The Handbag and Wellies Yoga Club

LUCY EDGE

EBURY
PRESS

1 3 5 7 9 10 8 6 4 2

Published in 2009 by Ebury Press,
an imprint of Ebury Publishing
A Random House Group Company

The Random House Group Limited Reg. No. 954009

Addresses for companies within the Random House Group
can be found at www.randomhouse.co.uk

A CIP catalogue record for this book is available
from the British Library

The Random House Group Limited supports The Forest
Stewardship Council (FSC), the leading international forest
certification organisation. All our titles that are printed on
Greenpeace approved FSC certified paper carry the FSC logo.
Our paper procurement policy can be found at
www.rbooks.co.uk/environment

Printed in the UK by CPI Cox & Wyman, Reading, RG1 8EX

ISBN 9780091930097

To buy books by your favourite authors and register for offers
visit www.rbooks.co.uk

For David

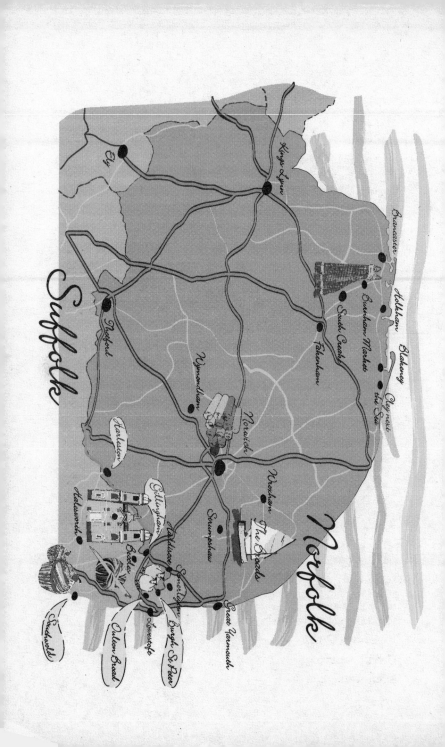

Contents

Author's note

I've changed some of the timelines in this book to help me tell my story with clarity.

I've disguised some places in this book to protect the identity of people who might otherwise be easily associated with them.

I've created some characters as composites and I've changed names and personal details for everyone, bar my family and those in the public eye. That's because no 'normal person' asks to be written about and it's fairer to separate them from my version of them, so that they are free to be the version of themselves they want to be. Hopefully my family love me enough to forgive me and, as for those in the public eye, well, they love it, don't they?

1

'Reincarnating hot water bottle covers with vintage cashmere'

I called them 'The Cappuccino Gurus' in honour of their unparalleled ability to dispense wit and wisdom over a frothy coffee. We met on a yoga holiday in southern Spain and now, seven years later, the four of us were the best of friends. Together we'd celebrated some seriously red-letter days – promotions, engagements, weddings and births – and we'd nursed each other through life's hard stuff: career burnout, serious illness and an assortment of toxic men.

Every Thursday night we gathered together for a yoga class, spurred on by thoughts of après yoga – a meal and several glasses of wine at Manna, the veggie restaurant opposite our local yoga centre. This hallowed ritual was the highlight of my week – I loved yoga but I loved The Cappuccino Gurus, Pinot Grigio and the restaurant's pistachio profiteroles more.

This evening I had something to share, something important. We settled into our regular table at the back of the restaurant, piling up our yoga mats in the corner. I studied the menu wishing, once again, that I was a yogic over-achiever – you know the type – the girl who parades around the changing room in a thong, showing off her sinewy fat-free limbs and washboard stomach. That girl would have no trouble choosing the Hijiki seaweed salad over the Mexican platter, the raw vegetables over the courgette fritters, the green tea sorbet over the pistachio profiteroles, but that girl was not me. The wine and wedges of crusty bread accompanied by lashings of rosemary-and-garlic-flavoured olive oil had barely touch landed when I made my announcement.

'Okay,' I said, trying to remember to breathe. 'Ladies – I have news.'

'Do I hear the patter of tiny feet?' asked Gabriele, a lioness of a mother who gave us, her three closest friends, the same fierce love as her two children.

'No, I'm afraid not,' I said, with a touch of sorrow – now *that* would have been great news.

'You're going travelling?' mused Poppy, running her hands through her mussed-up long blonde hair, exhibiting a youthfulness that had been forever preserved by the single act of marrying a man so much older than she. Now fifty, she looked like rock chick Pattie Boyd's younger sister. 'That's what I'd do if I was in your position – you've got the man, you don't have any children, you can do exactly as you please.' She sighed and twisted her haute hippy beads. 'I really envy your freedom – there are so many places I'd like to see – starting with South America – following the Inca trail, taking the train through Ecuador, dancing at Carnival, being the girl from Ipanema …'

Poppy's longing for freedom was understandable; her husband had promised more than he'd delivered and she, a gentle, sweet-tempered woman more interested in dreams than practicalities, had been left to raise the children and run their business more or less single-handed. Now that the children had left home and her divorce had come through she was looking forward to exploring those long-held dreams. I, on the other hand, had experienced enough years of freedom for one lifetime – I'd spent nearly a decade in the singleton zone and I had no intention of going back.

'Any more guesses?' I asked, directing my question at Andrea, noticing how well she looked; a bad break-up had been followed by a serious illness but, thanks to a brave heart, a lot of yoga and a newly acquired penchant for anti-oxidising broccoli, those unhappy days seemed to be far behind her.

'You and David got married?' she replied, blowing on her piping hot organic apple and cinnamon juice. 'You better not have done, I want to be chief bridesmaid – perhaps I'll marry the best man!'

'Come on, Andrea, we've only been together a year,' I said, giving her a pretend stern look, 'I'm forty-two and David's forty-seven, why rush to the finishing line?'

There were no more guesses and I couldn't contain myself another moment.

'David and I are buying a house in Norfolk!' I spoke into the silence of surprise. 'I'm trading my heels for wellies, my handbag for a trowel and this season's coat for a Barbour.' I paused, waiting for a response, and soon realised I needed to persevere in my effort to lift jaws from the floor. 'I know it's a bit of a shock, and I am really going to miss you all, but I have to do this now. I've spent twenty years working in advertising, putting my career first, and now I've met my man I'm going to make the most of it. And so, my friends, I've decided to take a year off; to get out of the rat race and put some time into what matters – settling down and starting a family.'

Gabriele was the first to respond. 'Have you found a place yet?' she asked; her own quest to find a nest for her brood had taken a year, but what a nest it had turned out to be – chaotic but warm and full of love.

We had. It was an old farmhouse just over one hundred miles from London, near a place called Beccles, a pretty market town at the southern tip of the Norfolk Broads – about twenty minutes inland from Southwold and half an hour south of Norwich.

'We're moving in at the beginning of July so we'll be able to enjoy the whole summer there. Imagine it: trips to the seaside, boating on the river, walking in the woods...' I sighed. I still couldn't believe my luck.

'And what's the house like?' asked Poppy, ever the interior designer.

'Let's just say it's a little more expansive than my pokey one-bedroom flat – there's enough room for the three of you to come and stay... you will come and stay won't you?'

'Of course we will!' replied Gabriele quickly. 'I might even bring my children... though you might wish I hadn't! They're being complete monsters at the moment.'

'Listen,' I said firmly, 'we've bought the house with children in mind and yours will always be especially welcome. We're even thinking of getting a gypsy caravan and putting it at the bottom of the garden – so if they're really badly behaved we'll just send them down there to sleep it off. What do you think?'

'A gypsy caravan? Don't give it to the children – I'll sleep there!' exclaimed Poppy, raising her hand in the manner of an eager child – a movement that resulted in a sudden cascade of jangling bracelets.

'It sounds great, Lucy,' said Andrea enthusiastically. 'You know I'm very tempted to come and join you – all that fresh air, good food, long walks, the ready availability of broccoli – so much more healthy than living in London.'

'Oh, please do, Andrea – come and be our neighbour, I'd love it.' Truth be told, the only thing I was worried about in moving out of the city was making friends – it would be so much easier to import my own.

'Perhaps when I find my man,' she laughed. There was a small pause. 'Do you mind me asking; was it a lot of money?'

'Actually the finances worked out okay – selling my London flat paid for half of the house, and David came into some money so that took care of the other half, and the cost of living is a little lower there – apart from the oil-fired central heating – so my savings will go further than in London.'

'You've always worked so hard,' said Poppy, 'all that time slogging away in advertising – don't feel guilty about it.'

'So, you're going to fill this house with children?' asked Gabriele, rubbing her hands with glee – there was nothing she liked more than a baby.

'That's the plan; picture me five years from now – an earth mother holding children's parties in fields of wildflowers, helping them collect shells and driftwood on undiscovered beaches, teaching them to sail on the Norfolk Broads...'

'Hmmm,' said Poppy dreamily, 'it sounds idyllic. Did you know that we used to go on family holidays on the Broads – we always sailed from Wroxham – perhaps we could take a boat out together in the summer?'

'That would be brilliant,' I laughed, 'my dad might join us – he's always fancied life on an ocean wave – or on a gin palace on the Norfolk Broads.'

'And how will you fill your days before the children arrive?' asked Gabriele, a woman whose own days were never less than full – aside from bringing up two children she was a well-known journalist in France and, despite the rough and tumble chaos that reigned at home, she was also working on a novel in her 'spare' time.

'Writing and leading the simple life – doing everything I can to look after myself, to nurture my inner fertility goddess, and I'll be looking after you too – watch out for Christmas hampers full of my home-made jam, mince pies and ginger wine. I'll tend my own vegetable patch, make cheese like Alex James from Blur, and I'll make my own clothes; I read about some American women who launched a successful business reincarnating hot water bottle covers with vintage cashmere.'

Everyone laughed; my home-making skills were not legendary.

'I'll be going for long walks, eating lots of fresh food, and,' I said firmly, contemplating the second glass of Pinot Grigio that I'd just poured myself, 'cutting down on my drinking – no more than three glasses a week from now on.'

'Perhaps you should think about giving it up completely,' said Andrea gently. 'I know it sounds tough but you *do* get used to it, and you'll feel so much better – it'll be almost worth the resulting social paralysis.'

'I hate to add my voice to the budding Temperance Society,' said Gabriele apologetically, 'but one of the women I met through my son's pre-school followed a hard-core fertility programme that required her, and her husband, to give up alcohol and coffee, use only organic cleaning products and follow an organic diet for six months. It all paid off – they had the twins three years ago, and now she's pregnant again. I can give you her number if you like.'

'I think that sounds too much like hard work,' said Poppy. 'You need to stay relaxed – don't over-think it.'

I was inclined to agree with Poppy but at least I'd already given up the coffee.

I'd developed a major Starbucks habit while I was working in advertising and kicked it with the help of *Dr Joshi's Holistic Detox* – a paperback I'd picked up in a second-hand bookshop for a pound – given that my caffeine habit had cost me half the national debt this had so far worked out to be a sensible investment.

'The move seems a good plan', said Gabriele, raising her left eyebrow slightly – a gesture that always betrayed a concern about to be expressed. There was a pause, then: 'It's just that it's such a long way from your life at the moment. I've always thought of you and David as Londoners – you love going out and having fun...'

'We do, and I'll really miss you all but I just need to get out of London,' I explained. 'I don't see myself getting pregnant here – we've been trying for nearly six months but it's not happening. I don't feel at home on the streets anymore and I think it might help to go back to my roots – I grew up in the Essex countryside, remember – so it's just a bit further north for me.'

'What about David?' joked Andrea. 'Has he ever left London before? Does he know where Norfolk is?'

'It'll be a bit more of a change for him,' I conceded. 'He did venture as far as Essex for university but he came back to London every weekend to hang out with his older brother at the Embassy Club, give his mother his washing and collect her food parcels. Anyway, that was thirty years ago and now he's as fed up with London as I am. He loves Norfolk too – he's got to know it from all the times we've stayed at my mum's house up near the coast. Don't worry – he's up for it.'

'So you will both be there full-time?' asked Poppy, refilling our glasses.

'I will, but David will keep his London flat because he needs to be in town to run his business.'

'I'm not being funny,' said Gabriele, 'but how are you going to get pregnant if he's here and you're there?'

'Booty calls, my dear!' I laughed. 'I have plenty of ovulation kits and I will take my temperature every day so as soon as it rises I'll jump in the car and head back to town – it's only two and a half hours away. It'll be fun – like being teenagers. And it won't be for ever, he's going to look at what it might take to run his company from Norfolk.'

'I think you're doing the right thing,' said Poppy decisively, dipping her fajita roll into a large dollop of guacamole – how did she keep her svelte figure? 'I must admit that I'm also thinking of leaving London. If I sell the house and the business I can buy a place in the south of France or Spain and set up a Boho yoga retreat.'

'That's a great idea!' we chorused.

'Would your new man come too?' I asked. 'Isn't he a property developer? Could be handy?'

'Maybe,' said Poppy hesitantly, 'I don't know where that relationship is heading at the moment but I do know that I don't really want to tie myself into anything right now – I'm just having fun. He's so much younger than me and I think he wants to settle down, start a family… I really don't want to go there again. Anyway, more on my plans another time – back to you, Lucy; when can we come and stay?'

'As soon as you like – it'll be your rural retreat – you can have long lie-ins and I'll cook breakfast for you, we'll go for walks and when it gets dark we'll retire for tea and crumpets in front of the roaring fire.'

'I'm so pleased for you, Lucy,' said Andrea, wistfully twisting a lock of hair round her index finger, looking like a lost teenager. The tremendous courage that had carried her through her illness seemed to desert her when it came to believing that she would ever find a man. 'You're what keeps me going when I've been on yet another disastrous date, you're my poster girl for happy endings over forty. I'm thirty-eight and I'm panicking – I read that a woman over thirty-five stands a one per cent chance of marrying, but here you are at forty-two; you've met your man, you're moving to the country and you're planning to have children.'

'Don't worry Andrea, it's your turn next,' said Gabriele, giving her a maternal hug. 'He's out there somewhere, and he'll find you – you've never looked fitter or happier or prettier – you're positively glowing these days.'

'You're intelligent and creative *and* you've got a social conscience – what's not to love, apart from your newly discovered penchant for broccoli?' I added, winking at her. 'I'm *sure* he's on his way to you right now. He probably just needs to tie up a few loose ends and then he'll be with you.'

Andrea smiled but didn't look convinced. I wished that I could magic up Mr Right for her – God knows I understood what it was to be single in your thirties when all around you were finding The One, settling down and having children. I had to hope that a change of fortune was just around the corner – she'd had such a difficult couple of years – but at least the experience had made her re-evaluate what was important in life. Thank goodness she'd plucked up the courage to leave that soulless job; she might've been a financial firector for a huge company but it made her miserable as sin. She was so much happier now that she was working for an organic cosmetic company, and the free samples that she liberally distributed to us (in the name of market research) were always a useful bonus.

We raised our glasses and Gabriele made a toast: 'To having it all in your forties.'

'And thirties,' said Andrea.

'And fifties,' added Poppy.

We clinked glasses and I tried very hard not to spill any of my Pinot Grigio – on three glasses a week every drop counted.

2

'Do not search for him, he will find you'

It was little wonder that I didn't find my man until I was forty-one. I was born a working girl, the best part of my childhood dedicated to building my career. As a nine-year-old my full schedule left little time for thinking about boys; I started the day with careful preparations appropriate to a secretary of my stature – selecting an outfit from my mother's wardrobe, making up my face, deliberating over the shoes – never the right pair. I spent my days answering the black Bakelite phone on my desk – 'Mr Baker is too busy to speak to you now. May I take a message?' – rearranging the notepads and pens I'd stolen from my father's office, taking dictation, choosing Mr Baker's new car for him as he was too busy to do it himself – it was always what I termed a 'honeybee' convertible – sometimes a Triumph Herald, but usually an MG Midget. The next thirty years played out pretty much as intended, except that I got to be Mr Baker.

My parents divorced when I was twelve and, as other children played outside the window, I spent a year hibernating in my bedroom seeking refuge in other worlds – my favourite book was Monica Dickens' *My Turn to Make the*

Tea about life as a trainee journalist – and I loved glossy magazines like *Honey, 19* and *Look Now*. By the time I'd graduated to *Cosmopolitan* and *Vogue* I'd settled on a career in advertising. Exactly what I would do in that world was by the by – the important thing was to be there, living a life inside those glamorous pictures had to beat lying on my Laura Ashley eiderdown reading about them. I toyed with a job in media buying – counting the number of pages of magazine advertising versus editorial content – then lines like 'Smitty did it', 'Fry's Turkish Delight... full of Eastern promise', and 'It's kind of new, kind of WOW – Charlie!' led me to consider life as a copywriter. I'd ask Mum for large sheets of paper so that I could lay out 'glass shattering' ads for Vivienne Westwood and Malcolm McLaren's black bondage suits.

Whatever the specifics of the job it was clear to me that I would need to move from the sleepy Essex village in which I grew up to London. All happiness lay in London. Sitting amongst the flowerpots on my stepmother Nikki's roof terrace I looked out over the streets of Fulham and determined that I would soon have my own open-plan sitting room, chocolate corduroy sofa and heated rollers.

By twenty-four I was a strategist at a top-ten ad agency on St Martin's Lane – now the site of the St Martin's Hotel (it tickles me that my then maroon and grey office is now a £300-a-night baroque bedroom with interactive light display). Imagine the thrill of working in the same building as the men who invented 'only the crumbliest flakiest chocolate tastes like chocolate never tasted before' and 'all because the lady loves Milk Tray', even if the ad I was working on was for McDonald's Neasden drive-thru. No matter, I was making money and, seduced by Paula Hamilton in that seminal 1987 VW ad, in time I bought the Golf convertible, the pearls, and the red bouclé wool suit with gilt buttons. I remained very single but I told myself, and my mum, that the mews house and the engagement ring would come later.

My life didn't revolve around marriage and children – in fact there were no children around. My brothers and sisters were all still at school or university, and my friends and I were taking time to find our places in the world. We were big kids in shoulder pads – life was about working, shopping, drinking and having fun, it was not about raising a family. When I stopped to think about it – which was never for very long – I couldn't imagine life as my mother. She had me at twenty-two – at that age I was staying late to check my secretary's typing or to run acetates through the photocopier. At thirty, when I was living on cigarettes and canapés, she was cooking for a family. By thirty-five, when I first toted a mobile the size of a brick around the wine bars of London, confessing details of my illicit office liaisons to friends and discussing the emerging World Wide Web with work colleagues, she'd divorced, remarried and acquired two stepchildren.

For a long time advertising's rewards were comparable to those of a good marriage – and a solid replacement for it – offering companionship and security, and as a **50% Extra!** bonus, challenging strategic problems concerning the fate of cartoon characters such as the Jolly Green Giant and the Vitalite singing sunflower. But there was an unfortunate side effect – as I progressed up the corporate ladder my love life slid down it. Where once, in my twenties, there'd been a lightness of touch in my office affairs (the odd snog and fumble behind the maroon and grey filing cabinet), by my thirties they were tarnished by the tinge of desperation. I might've dreamed of hand-held walks on Hampstead Heath, of returning to our house off the high street for tea and toast before a blazing fire, but my love life was, in the parlance of the time, 'a Gobi Desert'. My radar became increasingly attuned to emotionally unavailable men and I spent the few dates I did have feeling like someone catching a glimpse of what lay inside the cupboard of love but having the door slammed in my face before I could reach in and grab it. Instead of walking gracefully away, grateful to know what any viewer of *Sex and the City* understood beyond all reasonable doubt – that the only explanation for a man not asking you out, not wanting to come in for 'coffee', or not calling after a date, was that he wasn't 'that into you' – I'd get out an extra big chisel and try to prise the door open again.

My boss joked that my appalling love life was good for the company because I worked harder when I was in Man Misery. I blocked not having children out of my mind because they seemed to be a secondary problem – without a man they were never within reach. I didn't feel like I had any choice in the matter – but in reality it was what has been described by others as 'a creeping non-choice'. Focused on my career, Man Misery casting a long shadow over my desk, the possibility of a child felt so far away from me I just ignored it; so like all things ignored, it slunk away.

By the time I got to thirty-seven the career that had sustained me had burned me out. I was a group head in charge of a team of twelve, covering my own accounts and maternity leave for two other women. I didn't want to say no to the opportunity that I had worked so long to open up but I felt resentful towards these women – both of whom were on their third child. I picked up the slack but in so doing lost all sense of what was important in life.

Like the spinsters of the post-war years I was beginning to feel like a 'Surplus Woman'; without a place in the world I became brittle and increasingly isolated. I longed for someone to talk to, but work left me exhausted and with little time for friends. I was running on empty – I suspected no one would want to know me if they knew me well. Feeling that the friends I still had couldn't bear the weight of the way I felt I gave up, feigning happiness when I saw them, which was rarely. Like once big shiny balloons they gradually shrivelled away. I still got invited to the headline news – births, deaths and marriages – but I was no longer sharing the details of everyday life, the details in which I cried and wondered who I was.

I became addicted to American shows in which women met regularly, laughed and loved – I wanted to live on the set of *Friends,* and though I would never have admitted it in public, I envied Ally McBeal and the comfort of her always cheerful, sometimes fierce flatmate Renee. I longed for the quick-fire backchat of the *Sex and the City* girls, but mostly for the solidity of their friendship, the late-night phone calls, and the morning-after-the-night-before brunches.

My stepmother Nikki, who saw the mess I was in when I blubbed into my soup one evening, gently suggested that I might find yoga helpful, but it took the end of another barely off-the-ground relationship and a holiday in Tobago to persuade me to hit the sticky mat. There I witnessed a fellow holidaymaker spending the afternoons basking by the pool in a yellow bikini and baseball hat, quietly reading a yoga manual, and the early evening on the hotel lawn making bendy shapes with her pretzel-like body. Her graceful, soft yogic actions exuded peaceful vibrations that could be felt the world over and cast an unearthly spell over the male guests who ordered endless rum punches just to remain in her vicinity, and sat mesmerised, seemingly unable to speak or move. By the end of the holiday she had a boyfriend, and I had the name of her yoga teacher in London: Simon Low.

And so began the slow climb out of the hole that had become my life. Regular attendance at Simon's classes gradually lifted the albatross from my shoulders and helped me to peel back the layers of unhappiness, showing glimmers of something shiny and new – a gentle place where contentment might lie, a place where I could stop the striving, find out what would make me truly happy. Then there were the people I met along the way, especially the girls from that holiday in Spain; we were united in our unofficial quest – to peel back the layers that kept us from full expression of our best selves – and I finally stopped faking it. I had the friendships I longed for and together, the yoga girls I now knew collectively as The Cappuccino Gurus, helped me to confront the truth – advertising may have paid for the holidays and a steady stream of honeybee cars, but it wasn't nurturing my soul. Together we agreed that I needed to take a break from my career – take the maternity leave I needed to look after my own inner child. I took off for India and spent six months trailing round yoga schools, ashrams and eco-friendly villages with a shopping list consisting of the following:

Mystic Indian guru
Tantric bliss/sexual encounters

Pretzel-like body, flexible yet strong
Steady boyfriend, into yoga

Looking back on it I had a rather romantic notion that somehow, if I gave up my flat and my job, 'the universe' would provide the answers. This was a comforting thought, one that I shared with several single friends; I think our vague notions of the universe looking out for us and answering all the big and important questions on our behalves helped us believe we weren't alone. I placed my faith in its power to pick me up, guide me around India and settle me back down in the 'right' place, a place in which I would discover a new improved life. What I discovered was that the universe was not an 'other' thing; that I was very much part of it and as such, although it might help me along, ultimately I needed to take responsibility for myself. Suffice it to say, returning to London, I hadn't found any of the items on my shopping list but I was content to have discovered my Inner Guru – the teacher we all have inside us, the one with infinite wisdom, the one that believes *who* we are being comes before *what* we are doing or *what* we have. One problem. The Inner Guru turned out to be somewhat unreliable.

I tried a job in qualitative research but arriving in Manchester at five in the evening with the prospect of six hours of group discussions ahead of me, and the thought of The Cappuccino Gurus heading off to Manna without me, made me want to cry. No matter that I would be talking to normal people about their views on ads featuring a talking volcano or a new campaign to recruit maths teachers. No matter that I sat in a comfy Ikea-furnished sitting room in front of a huge pile of Marks & Spencer sandwiches and chocolate roasted peanuts. No matter that I returned to a boutique hotel at the end of the night, could order what I liked from room service, could lie comatose before a huge plasma screen TV, propped up by huge fluffy pillows. I took my mat with me but a glass of Pinot Grigio often won out over practising yoga with my feet pressed against the wardrobe and my nose tickled by dust under the bed.

I left research but unfortunately I still needed to pay the bills so, despite having cleansed my soul in the Ganges, I ended up back in advertising. At least I wouldn't have to work nights in Sheffield, I reasoned with myself as I got on the Tube with lead in my heart. I started off spending several weeks admiring the sparkling homes of premium dishwasher tablet users in the name of strategic development, and then I spent eighteen months Saving the World from Germs. I learned a lot about germs – although knowing that the cold germ can live on a door knob or a table for up to five days had me well on the road to developing a compulsive obsessive disorder – all I can say is, never touch the hotel remote control – worse, much, much worse, than dipping into the communal peanuts at the bar.

To my great surprise I really enjoyed working in an agency again, in part because the work was interesting, in part because the people were bright and, in the main, didn't take themselves too seriously, in part because I got to travel a lot, and in part because something inside of me had shifted. I'd learned from the so-called ordinary people I'd met in India that it was less about *doing* yoga – wearing a spiritual badge that implied certain lifestyle choices, including a predilection for green tea – and more about *being* yoga – seeing it as an aid to living, a way of living harmoniously with myself and other people. While I couldn't promise to *be* yoga all the time, or even some of it, I did want to try to increase the moments of seeing clearly and choosing wisely in everyday life, and that strategy seemed to work. I found a new appreciation for the small stuff – a frothy chocolate-topped cappuccino from the agency café, the global account director's 24/7 presence at the end of his BlackBerry whichever time zone he was in, the water cooler conversations regarding the previous night's episode of *The Office*.

I made the time to write and I loved sitting at my desk looking out of the French windows onto a balcony with views over a communal garden in which children played. The South Hampstead flat was only a few minutes' drive from Triyoga and aside from Thursday nights with The Cappuccino Gurus mostly I did my own yoga practice at home, 'upside downing' at sunset, just like the so-called ordinary Indians I'd met along the way. I felt more settled and happier than I'd been for years.

The one blot on the landscape was my Inner Guru's Male Toxin Radar, which was still suffering a serious malfunction. I'd met Mr Denmark in Chennai – he was a friend of one of my fellow students and he was hot. Hot. Hot. Hot. There was more than six foot of his strong tanned body, he had wide-set cornflower blue eyes and thick blond hair. I fell immediately in lust. I spent a long time convinced that he was The One – due to some unfortunate coincidences detailed in the Vedic astrology reading I'd had with Mrs P in Rishikesh.

Mrs P had said that I would meet a man 'into yoga and spiritual things'. Check: Mr Denmark was setting up a yoga centre in Copenhagen and counted Deepak Chopra amongst his closest friends.

Mrs P told me, 'He is not like you – he is older or not from your caste or not English.' Check.

Mrs P warned me, 'Do not search for him. He will find you.' Check. He'd found me on the beach in Mahabalipuram. It'd been, at least in my mind, a scene stolen from the movie *From Here to Eternity*, the surf rolling over us as we frolicked on the sand.

Mrs P said it would be a 'Love marriage. Good marriage.' This is where the prediction started to break down. Right after we'd finished playing Burt Lancaster and Deborah Kerr on the beach he'd told me, over a bottle of Tiger beer, 'I want a wife and family but I have issues around female dependency – my mother had a mental breakdown when I was seven and she was in hospital for a long time. Since then I am always the one to leave women.'

I should have jumped up there and then, wrapped myself in my sarong and run for the hills because, of course, he did leave. Some months later I spent a weekend with him in Copenhagen – I imagined us walking hand in hand, taking in the sights – the Tivoli Gardens, the Little Mermaid, the Viking Ship Museum... The reality was a little different. Mr Denmark drunkenly dumped me in a bar somewhere in the snow-bound city. I had no idea how to get back to his flat – which I wouldn't have bothered doing except that my passport was there. The next morning I got on the first plane home.

The Inner Guru really should have paid more attention to the small print of Mrs P's predictions – she'd told me I would meet The One after 17 February. I'd met Mr Denmark on 8 February. At the time I dismissed this as a small blockage in the cosmic information stream but clearly

I should've known better – Mrs P's 'black tongue' could speak no wrong.

I joined an old-fashioned matchmaking company and spent £400 on the privilege of one date – apparently no one else was compatible. 'You're at the top end of the acceptable age bracket – most of our gentlemen are looking for a woman in her twenties or early thirties.' He and I met at the Dorchester for a drink. He had oily fish eyes, more dependence on alcohol than even I could tolerate, and he was twenty years older than me. I told him I was going to the loo and jumped on a bus home.

Gabriele introduced me to a lawyer. I put his slow courtship – involving flowers and chaste kisses on the cheek – down to the fact that he was a perfect gentleman. Frankly I couldn't understand how we could get on so well and he could keep his hands off me until I heard, six months after I gave up on him, that he was gay.

By this point I had lost all faith in my Inner Guru Male Toxin Radar so I was quite happy to let Poppy's Inner Guru do the work – she wanted to introduce me to David, whom she'd met on another yoga holiday in Spain. She kept it low key, telling me she 'just thought we'd get on' and so, without worrying about it too much (something of a first for me), I agreed to meet him.

We arranged to go as a group to Ronnie Scott's in Soho where our friend Frances Ruffelle (a Tony award winner whom we'd met on another yoga holiday) was performing her favourite jazz standards and torch songs with the BBC Big Band. We'd celebrate Gabriele's birthday and I'd meet David. All well and good, until a couple of weeks before the gig I bumped into David at a Primrose Hill party. A cross between José Mourinho and the news reader George Alagiah, he had me at 'hello'. I sidled over to sit next to him but, when ten minutes later, he hadn't dropped everything to talk to me, I lost interest and left in a huff. I informed Poppy that I would be taking another man to Ronnie Scott's. She told me I should give David the benefit of the doubt, perhaps he'd been distracted by something, but my Inner Guru was resolute. No dice. He'd blown it.

Finally, in the queue to get into Ronnie Scott's with John, my replacement date, by my side, the Inner Guru spoke the first words of truth it had ever managed concerning men.

'You should be with him,' it said, sagely pointing at David.

Bloody hell. Now you tell me.

Fortunately John left early, citing depression and a headache. If David had been rude to me before he wasn't now – his manners were impeccable – he talked to me all evening (apart from when I was listening to John the Depressed), kept the champagne flowing all night and paid the bill at the end. Best of all, being of Indian extraction and into yoga he was one of the few people I could talk to about my trip round India without boring them to death. At the after-show party we found a quiet corner and exchanged 'how I got to where I am today' stories – he understood immediately the Inner Guru and her malfunctions, and even confessed to having had the odd malfunction of his own. He turned out to live round the corner from me in West Hampstead; only I could travel round India in search of a man only to find him ten minutes from home.

He rang me three days later, days that seemed to stretch into an eternity, and picked me up the following evening, opening the car door for me, driving to a candlelit Mayfair restaurant, paying for dinner and driving me home. I loved being out with him – an intelligent, handsome, confident, successful, grown-up man who called me 'Babe' – it might've been an old-school phrase but who cared? It made me feel young and sexy. I'd sit and look at him across the table, unable to believe my luck – his light brown skin glowing in the candlelight, his salt and pepper chest hair curling out of the top of his perfectly cut shirt. We talked about his business – an events marketing company – about my tour of India, about how life should be lived, and about yoga – debating the merits of Ashtanga (his choice) and vinyasa flow (mine).

I'd soon fallen for his sense of fun, his boundless energy for life and the way he came up with hundreds of ideas – often in one sitting. There was always a new project, a new scheme, a new way of thinking about a problem. He reminded me of that Kate Bush song 'The Man with the Child in his Eyes'; he had a child's endless enthusiasm and easy positivity, and when it was directed at me I felt I could do anything I wanted to do. I soon knew that life with this man would always be an adventure, and I found myself wanting to be there, by his side.

Much as I loved being out with him I loved being in the flat with him even more – his chest soon became my favourite place to rest my head and we spent many an evening on the sofa watching old films, lying together we were a perfect fit – as he said, 'you couldn't slide a piece of paper between us'.

Although our relationship had an air of inevitability about it from day one – several people at Frances's after-show party asked us how long we had been together – there were a number of what David politely termed 'considerations'. It turned out that we'd both built up some hard-to-lose habits in our combined years on this planet. Being with David wasn't always easy (and of course, he'd say the same about me) – he had such strong opinions on everything from yoga teachers and clothes to style and politics, just staying in the conversation could be a challenge – but as my mother said on meeting him, 'at least life will never be dull, dear'. Actually we disagreed about pretty much everything – what to eat, what to drink, what to watch on TV, how to drive, how to clean, how to cook, how to wash up – it could be exhausting, but when push came to shove, when I sunk into the heart of me he was there too, another root of the same tree.

We did, however, agree that it was time to buy a place together. We also agreed that it would need to be in a safe area and not be the size of a shoebox. There followed various ill-advised forays into unfamiliar territories – culminating in a dingy house on an A road with no central heating, few unbroken floorboards and walls that divided all of the windows in two. Its current owner had been renting out rooms as bedsits.

'It might be very useful to have a basin in every room,' I suggested.

'No, Babe,' said David firmly.

3

'Let's do it, Babe'

Actually there was something else we agreed on. We both wanted a child.

I'd kept thoughts of children at bay for so long that they took a while to trickle into my head. I started by imagining David as a father – the signs were good. He was great with his brothers' children and he even had quite an effect on children he didn't know – a little girl of three or four stopped in the middle of her walk on Hampstead Heath and stared at him, completely transfixed for several minutes, a one-year-old in her mother's arms was so keen to drink up every last drop of David that she cried when her mother turned away.

We began trying for a baby six months after we met. I'd spent all of my life trying to avoid pregnancy, so it seemed strange to be all of a sudden actively encouraging it. I woke up after the first attempt convinced the results had been instantaneous, protectively holding my belly in the super-market. As I cruised the aisles looking at baby food I allowed myself to notice other women with their children – a cohort I had effectively sliced from my visual map for many years, too painful to acknowledge. I was no longer irritated by the yummy mummies blocking the road as they parked their 4x4s in front of the nursery. I imagined myself walking down the Finchley Road heavily pregnant – thank God smock tops were in fashion. I imagined the warming smell of my baby's head, the tiny fingers and perfect fingernails. I imagined having a small hand to hold as I walked down the street. My world seemed to open up with possibility.

Now that I'd met my man and was trying for a baby, everything should have been cool and groovy in my world. So why was I feeling distinctly gloomy? I cast around for the source of my discomfort. It was London. I wasn't alone; the strain of living in the capital seemed to be getting to quite a lot of people – I read in the paper that 250,000 people had left it the previous year. I wasn't surprised – it was beginning to feel like one long piece of bad news – the suffocating silence of the Tube in the rush hour, the home-grown terrorists, the insane house prices, the congestion charge, the psychotic traffic wardens. David and I watched *Blow Up* and wished we could travel back in time to London circa 1966 – a time when even the parks were empty and you could park your car just about anywhere.

Everyone, including me, was angry – the motorist with a face twisted with rage because I hadn't reacted in the required nanosecond to the change in the lights, the young peacock on the Tube pushing past me as he pushed his jeans down so they barely held his buttocks, the woman behind me in the check-out queue who took my shopping off the conveyor belt when I popped to get a forgotten loaf of bread. For a second I wanted to slam her head into her precious guava fruit but I just about managed to contain myself, arriving home seething. This anger that I felt, this flash of need to have my presence on this planet acknowledged, seemed to be a collective emotion – one that was finding ever more extreme outlets in teenage knife attacks and gun crime.

We went on holiday to get away from the Angry City and to practise our new regime called 'let's have lots of sex and have a baby' (such was our dedication) but our post-holiday high was quickly punctured when we arrived back home to find a putrid smell in David's flat. An extensive search revealed a dead cat outside the back door – its leg savaged and crawling with maggots. I covered my face and cleared up with my plentiful supply of the leading brand of germ protection, blaming the foxes made native by a ready supply of domestic waste. The week got worse; a friend living in Mornington Crescent watched in horror as police removed a dead baby from a skip outside her flat. A headless body was found behind David's office, its fingers removed. I jumped off a bus and narrowly avoided being crushed to death by a twenty-three-year-old Bangladeshi girl – she jumped from the third floor of a council tower block round the corner from the flat, landing with an almighty crack no more than a metre away from me. The local vicar told me she was the fourth suicide in a fortnight – and the first one to survive. The ward sister told me she wouldn't walk again.

This city that I once loved was changing so rapidly it simply didn't feel like home anymore. It's ironic, and more than a little sad that, living in one of the world's richest capitals, I felt as if I was clinging to the bottom rung on Maslow's Hierarchy of Needs. Life in London had become all about survival.

Deciding that we needed to get out of town for the weekend we went to see my mum and Oliver, my stepfather, in Norfolk. They were appearing in their village drama group's annual pantomime – Mum's annual excuse to don thigh-length boots and a pair of bottom-skimming shorts and my stepfather's opportunity to wear boobs, a dress and more make-up than Jordan. This year it was *Pinocchio*. Mum's outfit took me by surprise – a full-length sparkling pale blue dress which she wore with a Marie Antoinette wig, also full of sparkle, and a sparkling wand – she was, of course, the Blue Fairy. Oliver was also out of his usual garb – I guess there were no pantomime dames in Pinocchio's village of Colodi and sadly neither the village policeman or the carpenter, both of which he played, were cross-dressers.

By the time I'd heard Mum's singing duet with Mr Cricket, the endless 'I'm inside a whale but I mustn't blubber' puns and the shameless plundering of the great classics 'Whale Meet Again' and 'Come On Puppet Light My Fire' – the horrors of London were beginning to recede. By the time I witnessed Mum's transformation from the Blue Fairy into Mrs Thatcher with the simple addition of a black handbag and an 'As I used to say to Dennis...' London had become another planet.

The next day David and I went for a walk to nearby Blakeney Point – we filled our lungs with icy air blowing in off the North Sea, enjoying the wide open space that came with the end of man-made things. The miles of salt marsh spread before us, we soldiered on, our bodies stooped against the abusive wind, our eyes watering and cast down towards the mud glooping and sloshing over the wooden boards that guided us towards steaming cups of tea and freshly caught crabs on the quayside.

On the way back to Mum's house, my pockets stuffed with home-made shortbread that I'd bought on the quay, we stopped the car to breathe in the soft sweet smell of sticky earth, to take in the stretching emptiness of the deep blue skies, the brick and flint cottages painted in the heritage colours of the National Trust, the flinty grey churches, the spiky washed-out yellow and red hedgerows that lined the road. Once again I felt a long way from London, a long way from the anger and desperation. Here, beneath this endless sky, there was a freedom seemingly absent from the Angry City. Here was an old England, the England of my childhood; Norfolk was protected by its isolation, a road to nowhere, a place of safety and certainty, a timeless place, a place to belong.

'I feel so at home here, David, so relaxed, so myself. I wish we could live here,' I said longingly. 'We could buy a farmhouse, grow our own vegetables, and raise some children.'

How else, when people were falling from the skies and cats were foxes' prey, was I going to become the fecund fertility goddess of my dreams – a poster girl for Earth Mothers everywhere? How else was I going to stand any chance of conceiving two beautiful children? (As David is such a handsome Indian I was hoping for Aishwarya Rai and Hrithik Roshan Bollywood look-alikes.) I imagined myself rooted in nature, receiving the healing potions of a reclusive ninety-five-year-old woman with a pointy chin and a hooked nose. She divines the precise moment of conception according to the traditions that have been passed down through generations of witchy healers and I am instantly with child.

'Okay,' said David.

'Sorry?'

'Okay.'

'But London is your spiritual homeland,' I said, panicking that my throwaway remark was about to change my life. 'What about your friends, your mum and sister, Ashtanga classes at Triyoga, all the restaurants…'

'Let's do it, Babe,' said David firmly.

And that was that.

Norfolk is a big county – the fourth biggest in England – encompassing more than two thousand square miles. Where to live? The obvious starting point was Burnham Market, just a few miles from Mum and Oliver. The self-styled 'loveliest village in Norfolk' certainly had plenty of charm: Georgian houses grouped around a traditional village green with some useful twenty-first-century embellishments – the deli, the local boutique hotel and Anna – the first in a small empire of luxe shabby-chic shops stretching all the way to Primrose Hill via Bury St Edmunds and Saffron Walden.

Three problems.

First problem: of course 'Chelsea on Sea' had Chelsea prices – we might as well have lived in London – and that wasn't taking into account the ruinous weekly bills I would surely run up at Anna in my quest to become sufficiently luxe shabby in my chic.

Second problem: there was something unreal, a little too perfect, about Burnham Market. It was almost a Hollywood interpretation of the perfect village – a backdrop against which a couple of thirty-something snowed-in sweethearts might fall in love. Truth was Hollywood had already been to Burnham Market – *Shakespeare in Love* had been filmed on Holkham Beach just up the road, a scene from *The Duchess* had been shot at Holkham Hall. My mother had landed herself a (small) part in this one, auditioning in the local church, getting in trouble for parking, along with hundreds of other hopefuls, in Tesco's car park.

Being an extra meant she wore a better-than-Botox eighteenth-century wig that pulled her forehead and cheeks in all the right places, and had to push up her boobs 'manually if necessary' just before 'lights, cameras, action!' The downside was that she had to plan to go to the loo long before she needed to as it took a while 'to excavate one's pants through the layers of petticoats'. During the breaks the female extras were given regulation white overalls and pink hair nets (the men had blue) to protect their eighteenth-century selves; so attired she tripped on her way to the refreshments tent (perhaps in too much of a rush for a sticky bun) and found herself looking up into the eyes of the young French chef. Unfortunately the doctor drove up on a scrunch of gravel before she could affect a full swoon – was he the fastest medic in the east?

Third problem: 'the loveliest village' was full of UFLs, 'Up from London' for the weekend, unable to believe their good fortune in discovering Anna on the north Norfolk coast. 'The fact is real people do actually live in the town and do their shopping here,' Mum grumbled as she narrowly missed out on a parking space to an SUV with London number plates.

She told us that she and Oliver had walked down the street behind a couple in matching Hunter wellington boots and Barbours, apparently up from Primrose Hill for the weekend. The country casuals had recovered from the excitement of seeing a branch of Anna but there was more to come. 'Darling,' cried the woman, stopping dead in her tracks, 'there's a *real* hardware shop!'

On another occasion Oliver popped into the fishmongers to pick up something for lunch. The queue was well and truly barged by a UFL in a hurry. She stood in the door and issued her instructions.

'Cooeeeee,' she shouted, getting the attention of the fishmonger and the whole queue. 'We're having a huge party tonight – we need lobster, smoked salmon – all that sort of thing. Just pop it all in the Jag will you – it's just outside. Got to dash.'

The Jag keys landed at Oliver's feet.

Nothing was said – but glances were exchanged.

Truth be told though, as Oliver said, there weren't actually that many people who could claim their first home was in Burnham Market. 'You can tell the number of second-home owners by the number of Yellow Pages left outside in their plastic bags. They are delivered on a Wednesday or Thursday and sit there until Friday night when they all come up.'

'This parish only has about 290 full-time residents out of 490,' said Mum gloomily. 'Sometimes I feel like an ethnic minority.'

These second homes only began to appear in the seventies when an increase in disposable income and city bonuses were matched to the number of empty homes in rural areas. 'That, plus better transport – think of all those eighties BMWs, Audis and Porsches tanking up the new M11 from the City – meant Essex and Suffolk got invaded,' explained Oliver. 'Okay, they may have run out of motorway long before they hit Norfolk but the pioneering spirit must've kicked in when they hit the county border, and that was enough for them to put up with getting stuck behind turnip trucks for an hour or two. Before that Burnham Market was,' he paused, choosing his words carefully, 'a dump.'

It had certainly witnessed some changes over the years, as Oliver remarked, 'older villagers remember using shire horses on the fields after the war and up until thirty years ago all the fruit was harvested by hand – fifty people would come and pick all the apples, nowadays it's just one or two.'

I have to admit that we did try following in the well-worn footsteps of our fellow UFLs – we had a brief flirtation with a barn in a hamlet so remote it took us several attempts to find it. The barn was unfinished – we told the land developer, a ruddy-faced man in a Barbour and traditional checked shirt, that we dreamed of turning it into a yoga retreat, using the stables as bedrooms. He seemed uncomfortable with our plans. 'I'm not keen on hippies,' he said, looking at me sharply. More than that he wanted 'to preserve the "Englishness" of the place', this time looking at David – perhaps even more sharply. No thanks.

We moved our search up to the seaside, tracking the coastline east from Brancaster to Cley Next the Sea. Would we find happiness in the lea of Cley's butterstone church, a church dedicated to St Margaret of Antioch? Perhaps her blessing as the patron saint of midwives would help us on our way to a joyful birth? Would a brick and flintstone with a path through the scratchy Brancaster dunes to the slate-grey sea be more our cup of tea? A cottage next door to the seventh Earl of Leicester at Holkham? I imagined Sunday morning walks through the ribbon of pine trees, emerging to the acres of sand, pebbles and driftwood, the water in the dim distant beyond, lying like a black pencil across the horizon. We could retire to the local pub to warm our wind-battered cheeks with a glass of red wine, some Brancaster mussels and estate-reared venison.

But in the end we decided that we didn't want to live somewhere so full of second homes, especially as it would effectively, for a year or two at least, be a second home for David. To paraphrase Groucho Marx, who wants to live somewhere full of people like you? David was quite clear on this matter, 'I want to live in the real countryside, where real people work and live.'

We spent hours on the Internet looking at what we came to call 'House Porn'. David was soon addicted to floor plans and thoughts of a wine cellar, and soon I was addicted too – unable to tear myself away from photographs of expansive farmhouse kitchens and walk-in fireplaces. Noticing that the price per square foot was considerably less in the east of the county we turned our attention to the Norfolk Broads. Having been on a barge holiday as a child I'd always had a soft spot for life on the water. Never mind that the holiday had ended in disaster; left to guard the boat while Dad and Nikki went to empty the 'honeypot' I was too enthralled with the twin pleasures of *Jackie* magazine's pictures of David Essex in a swimming pool and my Bounty bar to notice that the barge had drifted across the waterway, creating a boating tailback worthy of the M25 in the rush hour. Before I became an avid consumer of *Jackie* magazine I'd read rather too much Arthur Ransome, imagining myself as Dorothea having innocent adventures with Dick, sticky buns and ginger pop on the Broads. Now I imagined myself with our children on a *Coot Club* adventure, saving bird nests from egg thieves and from the unruly wash of motorboats owned by reckless 'Hullabaloos'.

We arrived in Wroxham – the place Poppy's family had used as a base for their boating holidays and the town from which Dick and Dorothea had set sail – as excited as a couple of nine-year-olds. But we were soon disappointed. Dick and Dorothea's concern for the preservation of their gaily painted sailing waters had proved well placed. Seventy years after *Coot Club* was first published the town was a shadow of its former self, sinking under the weight of so many motorboats that it'd been nicknamed the 'Clapham Junction of the Broads'.

As Clapham Junction was one of the reasons we were leaving London we switched our search to the southerly reaches of the Broads. The area was not as chichi as north Norfolk, in place of the winding lanes and pretty unoccupied flint stone cottages were straight roads bordering endless fields, fields sparsely populated with huge built-for-purpose farm buildings and wind turbines. It was closer to London – and equidistant between Mum and Oliver, and Dad and Nikki who live in north Essex. We soon found a traditional farmhouse on one of our favourite house porn sites that looked interesting – it backed onto farmland and woods and faced fields full of sheep.

We drove up from London one Saturday morning full of excitement. We wanted to explore the town first, to get a sense of the place, before driving to the farmhouse a few miles away. We passed a vast Morrisons and Tesco, which made us feel dispirited and relieved at the same time. We stopped to admire the colourful carved sign that portrayed Queen Elizabeth I presenting the Royal Charter to John Bass, the first Portreeve (like a mayor but with more responsibilities) of Beccles in 1584. We drove around the centre of town looking for a parking meter but there were none – nor were there any draconian traffic wardens ready to harass us – in fact, the only restriction on the free parking was a two-hour limit so, not quite believing such a thing was still possible, we parked by a massive sixteenth-century bell tower, continuing to look back at our still-untowed car with disbelief.

Detached from the main building of St Michael's the tower looked somewhat marooned – apparently at 3,000 tons it was deemed too risky to put it in the normal position because the rest of the church was on the edge of a cliff – we couldn't work out if this was an accident or by design. Climbing the ninety-nine-foot-high spiralling staircase we stood at the top taking in the view – despite the murkiness of the day Beccles' old-world charms were immediately apparent in the patchwork of rooftops and Dutch gables, in the narrow streets lined with Georgian houses and in the market square, where shoppers were taking time to stop and chat. Looking out to the west we understood how Beccles, which means 'meadow by the water', had acquired its name. We admired the eight-berth cruisers and canoes on the River Waveney down below, shivering as we watched them bravely slicing through the clean dark water that formed the watery border between the two counties; Norfolk's open marsh-lands and meadows, and our farmhouse, lay on the far side of the river, the pretty riverfront houses of Suffolk lay on the nearside, on a quaintly named street called Puddingmoor.

Back down on earth we walked around the town, each of us finding our own pleasures – David got very overex-cited about finding a wool shop where he could get his jumpers mended and became positively delirious when he found a gunsmith's and licensed game dealer. He went in to talk clay pigeon shooting with the check-shirted gentleman with the handlebar moustache, while I looked in on the busy library with its notice board covered in recruitment ads for the Girl Guides, rotary club, WI, bowls club and Morris dancing. We met again in front of the smart façade of the local deli – deciding it would be a useful antidote to Tesco. We took a break in bustling Twyfords, converted from an old gentleman's tailors established in 1919, munching on toasted teacakes surrounded by glove drawers, wooden changing screens and the still smartly turned-out people of Beccles. Finally the clock pulled up at half past two, it was time to go and see the farmhouse; our stomachs fluttering with excitement, we emerged from the teashop pulling on our coats and putting on our hats – it had begun to rain.

We headed out of town along the main road, passing signs to a village hall and another church. Pulling off into a succession of narrow lanes we rounded a final sharp bend, drove through a post gate and up a gravel drive, admiring the lanterns marking the corners of the farmhouse that rose up out of the gloom and parking to the side of a large willow tree, glistening in the rain.

Standing to attention at the front door of the pretty house with a French pantiled roof was a retired army man wearing a check shirt, mustard cords and sporting a well-trained moustache. We shook his hand, establishing in the initial introductions that he was a 'Saturday boy' for an estate agent and that the owner was away but, knowing that we'd had a long journey, had said to make us feel at home. He took us round the side of the house and we walked through the back door into a big country kitchen with an old cooking range, a worn refectory table and ladder-back chairs.

A chewed-up dog basket sat in the corner, a row of china pigs adorned the mantelpiece, frogs leapt from tile to tile. David busied himself inspecting the chewed-up knobs on the lower level cabinets, intently opening and closing drawers. I stood at the butler's sink and looked out at the garden, it was wildly overgrown but beneath the brambles I could see the thorns of dormant rose bushes. Would David propose to me one hot summer's day, getting down on one knee amongst the roses? Beyond lay an open expanse of lawn – just big enough for a marquee – perfect for a wedding reception. David came over and put his arm round me, pulling me close – was he thinking the same thing? I was dying to know but I didn't dare ask, didn't want to risk spoiling my dream. One thing was clear – this house already had us both firmly in its grip.

The 'Saturday boy' made himself scarce, leaving us to walk round the rest of the house together, hand in hand. We stood in the doorway of the sitting room taking in the large room packed with overstuffed sofas, the black baker's oven and the heavy scorch marks on the beam above the walk-in fireplace. We looked out over a farmhouse track, an old barn and a distant house, smoke curling out of its chimney, lights making a home out of the dusk. Treading gingerly now, for fear of discovering something that would destroy our dream, we moved through room after room filled with the clutter of family life: a doll's house in a bedroom, a flotilla of yellow rubber ducks in a bathroom, a collection of teddy bears in a cupboard. We surreptitiously inspected the photographs of children and dogs that covered every surface.

We were soon plotting what to do with each of the rooms. Which bedroom would make the first nursery? Where would the cot go and what colour would we paint the walls? We stood at the window of what we'd decided would be our bedroom and looked out over the willow tree and fields, the lights from a clustering of small houses and what might be a village hall half a mile away, St Michael's tower dimly discernible in the distance.

We borrowed some wellingtons from a pile by the back door, venturing into the fast-fading light. The lanterns on the sides of the house illuminated a haphazard row of trees, hinting at what might once have been an orchard, a waterless pond revealed its torn plastic lining, a run-down stable block – could it become a yoga studio? We took a short walk along muddy farm tracks towards the hundred-acre wood behind the house – would our children find Christopher Robin and Kanga there? It was getting too dark to make out any more than the ragged outlines of sycamore trees so we turned back shivering, pulling our collars up against the chill wind.

Gratefully we returned to the warm fug of the coffee-scented kitchen, sat at either end of the long table and pretended to have breakfast.

'I say, Lucy, would you pass the toast?' said David, in his best accent.

'Darling, would you be a dear and pass me the *Telegraph*?' I countered.

We looked at each other and laughed.

Four months later, at the beginning of July, we moved in.

4

'We make barbecue for you'

Within hours of moving into the farmhouse a lifetime's accumulated junk had been unboxed and arranged – admittedly the contents of my pokey London flat didn't exactly fill the house, but it fitted right in. If only the same thing could be said about me… A few weeks later I still had some adjusting to do.

There were no headless corpses or knife crimes in Beccles – instead young men were arrested for driving too fast, breaking shop windows, stealing bicycles, and throwing chips at each other. There were no foxes savaging cats in Beccles. They'd all moved to West Hampstead in search of an easy life. There were no tower block suicides. This was in part because there were no tower blocks, but also because no one jumped anywhere, or even ran.

It seemed as if Beccles (population 9,746) was on a permanent go-slow. Although the self-styled 'small town with the big heart' had recently acquired a Laura Ashley and a WHSmith, most of the shops were a little more homespun, preserving some of the character of the town that must've existed in the thirties when a young woman who worked as a shorthand typist at Messrs Clowes and Sons, where they printed millions of copies of Beatrix Potter and the Bible, could spend her Saturday buying bread from Tooks the baker, browsing Miss Lockwood's selection of ribbons, paying tuppence to watch the Regal's matinee double bill *The New Adventures of Tarzan* and *Tarzan and the Green Goddess*, and buying a crème de menthe half cornet from Mr Pitkin's Ice Cream Parlour to lick on the way home. We still had Delf's Garage (established 1856), Robert Tilney the aforementioned gunsmith (established 1860), Seppings the butcher (established 1918) and two sixteenth-century coaching inns in the market square, but sadly the five 'bottle and glass' shops that operated from back rooms in Northgate had long since closed up, the old cinema had been turned into a pizza place and Tesco now occupied the site of the printing works. Perhaps the biggest shame was that Tooks, the town's artisan baker, had never been replaced – one day, wearing his customary white overalls, the baker had found himself in an early morning blizzard and was knocked down by a horse and cart made silent by the snow. Who'd have thought that the production of sticky buns could be so dangerous?

These days the town's streets played host to three key demographic groups – pregnant women, mums with young children and grey-haired seventy-somethings. The demographic profile of the town was played out in the *Beccles and Bungay Journal* classifieds; there were some single mums seeking 'fit and active' men in their thirties, but there were a lot more 'young at heart' older ladies. I wondered if the seventy-eight-year-old widow with hazel eyes who liked 'bowling, days out, coast and drives' had teamed up with the 'slender gent' of seventy-six who was seeking 'an ordinary lady who likes dancing, trips to the seaside, walking and country life'. Sounded like a perfect match to me.

We were quick to appreciate what we had – the ladies in the wool shop who darned David's jumpers at three pounds a pop, Twyford's perfect cappuccinos, Sepping's award-winning sausages, the exacting car maintenance at Delf's ('I'm a newcomer,' said mechanic Joe, 'I've only worked here fifty-two years') and the girls in Fresh and Fruity, the local greengrocer – but we never got out of these shops without spending time as well as money. There was always at least one sentence about the weather, and more often than not one sentence led to another and before you knew it ten minutes had gone by before you'd finished catching up on the salient points of the day. I wanted to love the chat and I tried really hard to appreciate the fact that I no longer had to use anger to persuade others of my existence – but that first month was characterised by a fizzing impatience as my body clock struggled to adjust to the time difference in what felt, at times, like a different country.

I was driven slightly mad by the number of people calling unannounced at the farmhouse. Every time someone knocked at the door I lost at least an hour to 'mardling' – the Norfolk term for a leisurely chat. Not every conversationalist was entirely reliable – sitting at our kitchen table I heard that one of the local houses had been a suspected IRA safe house – why else would the family who moved in need six removal lorries and be guarded by Gurkhas? I heard that our sitting room was once a cowshed – with an original fireplace? I heard that we were setting up 'a yoga commune'. I heard that there was a bricked-up doorway concealing a secret passageway that once linked our cellars to an inexhaustible supply of brandy, tobacco and tea, smuggled down the River Waveney from the North Sea. I heard that the secret passage could be traced by the hollow sound a horse would make in riding over it. I heard that our farmhouse was haunted by the ghosts of smugglers. I tried to relax into the intrigue, to enjoy the Chinese Whispers, but twenty years in advertising had left me so hardwired to deadlines and solid facts that the effort of sitting still and dealing in hearsay left me breaking out in a cold sweat.

I may have been only two and a half hours from the stresses of London but I was still running on London time; I envied the skylark's ability to climb unimpeded into the summer sky as I got stuck behind caravans laden with bicycles making their slow way up the A143 towards Great Yarmouth. It was just as slow in the opposite direction – I went to the local museum and learned that the first stagecoach had journeyed from Beccles to London in 1707 – I wondered if, more than 400 years later, the road was any faster. Watching our oak-tree incarnate gardener plant grass seed with his digger-bucket hands, I asked him why it didn't grow more quickly. When he stopped pulling out tree stumps to have a cup of tea and discuss the recently sprung blooms, did I stop and smell the roses? No, not me. I had places to go, phone calls to make.

I went for a lot of walks that July, partly to get some exercise and partly to slow down. I'd leave by the back gate and not see another soul until I got back to the farmhouse – if the same thing happened in London I would've had to assume that a nuclear bomb had gone off. I'd nod to the ducks in the pond and the white barn owl, or 'old hush-wing' as owls were called locally, perching on the fence, walk briskly across a field filled with wheat and past a fairy tale house which could've been the children's home in Enid Blyton's *Enchanted Wood*. From here I'd round the corner into the woods, take a deep breath to inhale the musty smell of cowslip and the dusty track, taking care to avoid breathing in the midges, watch the pheasants and hares scattering ahead of me, trying to be soothed by the soft cooing of the woodpigeon, the darting of tiny yellow butterflies and the gossamer wings of hundreds of dragonflies.

The peace, the smell of fertiliser, the huge flat landscapes broken only by grain storage silos and a church, all of these things should've taken me a long way from London but I spent the thirty-one minutes it took to complete this circuit thinking about all the things I needed to do when I got back to the house. Sometimes I even rode my bike so I could do my daily walk faster. Now there was nothing but a year of freedom and relaxation before me I felt guilty and anxious. I filled up the days with tasks – food shopping in Beccles, making beds, registering with the doctor, weeding the garden, planting herbs, combing the charity shops for cashmere jumpers to reincarnate into hot water bottle covers. I began to have a minor identity crisis – without the goals and deadlines that came with Saving the World from Germs then who was I? I realised that I was, like James Joyce's Mr Duffy, 'living a short distance from my body'.

I couldn't settle so I decided to pay London a visit. Even in that short space of time – barely a month had elapsed since the big move – it seemed that much had changed, principally my attitude to the city. David and I spent a sunny afternoon on Marylebone High Street, browsing the Edwardian oak galleries of Daunts bookshop, trying out huge sofas with matching price tags in the Conran Shop, eating at our favourite restaurant. I enjoyed the familiarity of the London streets, the friendly but distant shop assistants, the diversity of race and the anonymity; no one wanted to get to know me, and no one wanted me to get to know them. I realised that in Norfolk I'd felt as if I were living under a microscope – examined to see what box I fitted into, given an identity that would, if I wasn't careful, become a straightjacket for years to come. We'd been advised that 'there was an "us" and a "them"', that there was 'a line we shouldn't cross', that we shouldn't have workmen sitting at our kitchen table, that we shouldn't make them cups of tea, much less give them a biscuit. We ignored the advice, it wasn't our way of doing things, but we had yet to navigate a new course that would allow us to be friendly without losing hours to the mardle. Back in London I breathed deeply, gladly filling my lungs with pollution and the freedom that comes with a Londoner's ability to own multiple identities, travel across different groups and share a cup of tea with whosoever they chose.

That Thursday night I joined The Cappuccino Gurus for some yoga and the usual table at Manna. It felt good to be back, to do a class together, and to air my frustrations.

'Do you think maybe, just maybe, you've been rushing things a little?' asked Andrea, tucking into her organic roasted beetroot salad. 'Think about it logically – how can you expect to have grown roots in those fields when you've only been there a month?'

It wouldn't be the first time I'd rushed at something; 'I suppose I've only just, as the locals would say, "blown in",' I conceded. 'The owner of the local bookshop told me that he's still regarded as a "blow-in" even though he's been there twenty years; by those standards, I've got a way to go.'

'It's not going to take you twenty years, Lucy,' said Gabriele, putting her hand on mine. 'Just give it a bit of time; you'll make some friends soon, I'm sure.' She disappeared outside for a cigarette.

'Gabriele is right,' I said, firmly biting down on another Edamame bean. 'I guess the adjustment period is bound to be a bit lonely. Maybe if I was already pregnant I'd be feeling better about things and of course I'd be meeting plenty of other women in the same boat – the streets of Beccles are packed with pregnant women – it's all baby boots, or granny boots.'

'You'll be okay, Lucy,' said Poppy, adjusting the collection of paisley print scarves at her neck. 'I *know* you're going to have children.' As her matchmaking had bought three couples to the altar, and her sister was a white witch in Devon, her instincts were to be trusted. 'And didn't that fortune teller in Rishikesh tell you that you would?'

'No, I'm afraid she didn't,' I said regretfully, remembering Mrs P with affection. It was the only subject she'd been vague about, enigmatically telling me 'you will decide'. It was the taxi driver who said I would – though he was wavering about the numbers. The closer we got to my destination, and his tip, the larger the predicted number of children.

'Lucy – honestly, get real! You've got to give all that healthy air a chance to work!' said Andrea firmly, pouring me some water.

'I know, I'm just worried I might be leaving it rather late,' I admitted, staring into my glass, 'but I guess plenty of women do it in their forties – Madonna, Halle Berry and Jerry Hall all had children at forty-one.'

'The woman who plays Bree from *Desperate Housewives*

was forty-four and Helen Fielding was forty-eight,' added Poppy, curling her perfectly formed frame into the back of her chair. 'Obviously it's possible.' I wondered, once again, how that tiny body had carried two children without any evidence of ever having been stretched beyond eight stone.

'It's all about your state of mind – it will happen, just keep positive,' said Andrea, 'that's what worked for me when I was ill.'

'And remember, we're right behind you; if you need any help, or numbers, just let us know,' added Gabriele, returning from the cold night, removing her perfectly tailored red wool coat and wafting the faintly decadent scent of strong French tobacco across the table. 'There are lots of older mums with children at pre-school – I can ask any of them for help or advice *if* you need it, which you won't.'

By the time Andrea's vegetable tagine and our Mexican platters had arrived all faith in my mission had been restored. I would stay relaxed and do the things I loved to do and everything else would surely follow.

We moved on to Andrea's love life. She'd been on a disastrous date with an Albanian building contractor who'd been refurbishing her company offices.

'He turned up reeking of aftershave, attempted to snog me within twenty minutes and announced that I was the woman he'd been waiting for all his life,' she said, exasperated. 'I managed to last a couple of hours but in the end I had to run away – then he called me at least fifteen times over the course of the weekend.'

'Have you tried *Guardian* Soulmates yet?' I asked. 'I answered an ad on there and met a handsome book illustrator.'

'What happened?' asked Andrea, excited at the prospect of a new door opening.

'Sadly, there was more chemistry in our glasses of Pinot Grigio than in our body language,' I admitted, 'but that shouldn't stop you – he was *very* handsome.'

Andrea promised to give it a look, along with match.com, which, she'd heard, was offering a money-back guarantee.

I wished her all the luck in the world – I was so glad I was out of the dating scene, so grateful that I had found David, and all I wanted was for my friends to find love too.

Poppy was feeling exhausted. 'It's my young man – we're out clubbing or hanging out at one of his friends' houses almost every night. It's all right for him, he's got the kind of job where he can sleep in until ten but I have a business to run. I fell asleep in a bar last night – the sofa was so comfortable I just curled up and before I knew it he was waking me up to go home…'

'Because he could see you were exhausted?' Andrea asked.

'No', said Poppy sorrowfully, 'because the place was closing.'

'You should definitely try an older man,' I suggested, 'mind you, David is five years older than me and he never gets tired – he doesn't even need to drink; while we're all talking nonsense at three in the morning he's running on coffee – as long as the bar does a soya latte he's happy.'

Poppy moved on to her continuing interest in creating a boutique yoga hotel – she was torn between Spain, Italy and the south of France.

There was a general consensus that she'd make it amazing wherever it was.

'Can you do anything about the snoring roommates and

the communal bathrooms?' I asked. 'We all love yoga holidays but they can come with some significant challenges...'

'Don't worry,' replied Poppy, ever the haute hippy; 'I'm thinking single bedrooms with ensuite bathrooms, Zoffany linen walls, Peruvian alpaca wool bedspreads...'

'Hand-blown glass bowls filled with white sand from the healing beaches of Byron Bay?' quipped Andrea, who'd spent a happy three months acquainting herself with the cream of eastern Australia's surfers and yoga teachers when she was convalescing from her illness.

'Sacred Tibetan tree bark sculptures?' I added, pouring myself a second glass of Pinot Grigio. 'Or perhaps they could come from Norfolk? There are some really beautiful trees in our woods...'

'Actually, a good night's sleep would be enough of a luxury,' said Gabriele mournfully. She was struggling with the realities of raising her young children; her husband, though keen to help when around, was not around – his job kept him at his desk from eight till late. She was also wrestling with the competitive world of north London parenting.

'It's appalling,' she opined. 'The children aren't free to be children, their achievements and activities are traded as social currency – it's as socially differentiating as where you live and what car you drive. Failure to send Tarquin Superbus to at least one activity per day – choose from football, judo, swimming, music, French, Mandarin, ballet and athletics – results in social ostracism. Some children even "play" once a week with a tutor,' sighed Gabriele. 'What's wrong with children playing with their friends?'

'Perhaps you should move to Norfolk,' I suggested hopefully, 'it seems to be much more relaxed up there.'

'If only we could, Lucy,' said Gabriele. 'I could do some of my work from Norfolk but unfortunately Pierre's job keeps him in London and I can't separate him from his children, or me – I just don't think it would be very good for our relationship.'

I knew what she meant. I was finding being apart from David during the week pretty hard work – I really missed him and, even though I would still count myself as being on London time, it often took a while for us to tune into the same wavelength when he came back from the Angry City. Well, we'd have to see what happened – right now I just needed to focus on staying relaxed.

I left Manna feeling much more myself. Talking through my issues and listening to the Gurus had taken me back to a place I could call home – these were normal dilemmas, not involving cogitations on the subject of ghosts, smuggling or IRA safe houses, these were conversations in which I knew my contribution would be valued and acknowledged. These conversations were the bread and butter of my emotional life.

Returning to the farmhouse, via a slow train that seemingly stopped at every village between London and Beccles, I put my energy into nesting; David was taking care of the exterior – fixing the roof and repointing some of the brickwork – so I focused on the interior. Looking at the empty spaces it was clear that we needed some furniture; the entire contents of my flat fitted into the house's sitting room. Norfolk and Suffolk have fantastic antique shops in every direction but they also have fantastic prices and I ended up feeling like Hans Christian Andersen's little match girl – pressing my nose up against shop windows and dreaming of the day when I would be invited in to share a roast goose at the mahogany table decorated with silverware and huge candlesticks.

Meanwhile, back in the real world... I enjoyed my trip to the local auction house where I perused treen wig powder shakers, crown pin cushions and nineteenth-century copper jelly moulds in the company of a curious mix of Arthur Daleys and toffs in mustard cords. After a break for a piping hot mug of tea and a sausage roll I found the energy to buy a Royal Horticultural Society garden bench, a pair of church pews and a slightly wonky chair, for a total of £100. Feeling rather pleased with myself I informed David of my purchases – he didn't realise we needed these things and asked whether they had a returns policy. Undeterred I took the wonky chair, and an armchair that a friend of Mum's gave us, to the upholsterer who said the wonky chair was irreparable but he'd take forty pounds off the price of upholstering the armchair because he could use the wonky one's castors. Lesson learned I stuck with John Lewis, and David came with me. Always one to sniff out a bargain he'd take their sale price and offer them half. The first time he did this I was embarrassed – negotiating with John Lewis felt like asking the Queen if you could take home a souvenir from Buckingham Palace – it just wasn't done.

'Relax, Babe,' he told me, 'I've got suits half price from Harrods – they need the business, just watch.' I relaxed, and he triumphed, always. I have subsequently tried it myself – let's just say there's something in his technique I'm missing.

Poppy came for a weekend to relax, and to give us some decorating advice. Seeing her in our sitting room was like having a favourite armchair returned – her presence helped to make the place our own. After some much-needed lie-ins (she was still dating the younger man), some long luxuriously scented baths, some walks in the woods – which she did wearing a pink kaftan and silver wellies – and some excursions to the local pub, where her unique brand of Boho glamour attracted the attention of all the men, she was ready to give us her wisdom, starting with paint colours. As a highly respected interior designer whose work has featured on the covers of *Elle Deco* and *House and Garden* we trusted her taste, but we were a little nervous – Poppy may have been a wonderfully whimsical confection when it came to her friends, but she didn't mince her words when it came to giving her professional opinion. She'd walked through every one of the three rooms in David's London flat and concluded that 'the least offensive room' was the white-tiled bathroom.

She walked through the farmhouse wrinkling her gorgeous little nose, swirling her washed silk skirts, jangling her golden bangles and pronouncing the Farrow & Ball colours that spoke to her. We followed. I took notes.

The hall?

'Pigeon.'

The library?

'Hardwick White.'

The sitting room?

'Parma Gray.'

We had a good giggle about the names of those paints – Hardwick White was actually grey, Parma Gray was actually blue, House White was actually yellow. No matter. We knew what was needed and, thus armed, we went about trying to find some local painters – it was too big a job for us. One problem: we didn't know where to look for local painters.

'Don't worry, my love,' said David. 'I'll get Bruno to do the work. He can live up at the house while we are on holiday and blitz it.'

Bruno was David's Polish builder in London. He was a large and helpful man who'd developed a huge crush on Poppy when she'd had him over to build her a new wardrobe. The job had taken rather longer than was strictly necessary but he had waived all charges in a fit of generosity of which we'd never been the beneficiaries. He had, however, built David a wardrobe, installed a new kitchen and painted all the walls in his flat in the space of a fortnight. He was very enthusiastic about the idea of a month in the country, though I must confess I might've told him Poppy was going to be popping in. Secretly I worried for him – how would he fare in the windy reaches of east Norfolk? Would he be able to get hold of Polish food? What would he do for company? Would he be lonely? I hoped that he might bump into some of the 60,000 Poles already living in East Anglia – they were mainly working in agriculture so perhaps he'd meet one on the neighbouring farm.

I needn't have concerned myself. He established himself very quickly; when we arrived back at the house the TV was thumping with MTV Base, two extremely large men were banging away in the library and two women sporting cleavage-boosting T-shirts, gold hoop earrings, vertiginous heels and sprayed-on stonewashed jeans were in my kitchen. I went to the fridge to deposit my half-pint of semi-skimmed milk but there was no room – it was full of giant Lukullus Juniper sausages, U Jedrusia dumplings, and yogurts, so many yogurts.

Bruno arrived back from Morrison's with several hundredweight of sausages, some tinned eels, and a red face.

'Hello, David. Ah – I have been naughty boy. I not tell you I ask our sisters to stay. No problem?' he asked hopefully.

To my surprise David was quite laid back about this. At least until he realised they'd been doing some of the painting.

'Bruno, we are paying you to do a professional job, this is never going to happen again. Do you understand?' said David firmly.

'Yes, David. Never again. We make barbecue for you?'

This is how we came to have a Polish barbecue in our back garden. It was a hot August night and it involved many large burned on the outside, raw on the inside sausages, some eels and a lot of yogurt. Madonna thumped on the iPod, the boys and me sat and drank cheap beer from the bottle, watching the sisters dance their way round the garden; I tried to appreciate the way they were aerating the lawn with their heels.

The next morning David and I left to go into Norwich – when we returned that evening there was no sign of the Poles, their tools or their Lukullus Juniper sausages. David rang Bruno and was told that his mother had been critically injured in a car crash and they'd flown to Poland to be by her bedside.

We never heard from Bruno again. If you see him please ask him for the advance we paid him.

It was clear we needed to find some locals – we might fare little better but at least they would go home at the end of the day – sometimes at three in the afternoon, we were told. But where to find them? Enter Dom Antony Sutch, a Benedictine monk who'd been a chartered accountant and headmaster of Downside School before becoming Beccles' parish priest in 2003. I'd heard him speak on Radio Four's 'Thought for the

Day' and was keen to meet him – in fact it was this, rather than any religious fervour on my part, that got me to church in the first place. David, being a good Catholic, would've gone whoever was in charge. Reasoning that Dom Antony would know most of Beccles, or at least the Catholic bits, we asked him, at the end of service one day, if he knew anyone who could help us find some reliable people to help us effect a smooth transition to the countryside. In the end his list amounted to a list of one – but what a name it was.

She swept up our drive one Sunday. I saw her feet first – a fabulous pair of bronze Birkenstocks glittering in the sun as they emerged from the Range Rover. I thought that we would probably be friends. Then the rest of her emerged – a fifty-something perfectly coiffed auburn-haired beauty clutching a bottle of Dom Perignon. Yes, we would definitely be friends.

Lady Birkie turned out to be a fabulous blend of mother hen, networker and fixer par excellence; she spent two hours in our kitchen kindheartedly downloading the entire contents of her address book. I spent the entire time ruing the fact that the kitchen was cold and the cupboard was bare. She politely soldiered on, fuelled by no more than several cups of Earl Grey tea, not complaining that she was spending Sunday lunchtime freezing and starving to death when she could be in her own kitchen cooking up a feast for her husband and four children. Not only did she give us the names of the only carpenters, plumbers and painters worth knowing, she also took hold of my fledgling writing career with a very firm grip.

Such was her talent she could so easily have followed in the footsteps of Lynne Franks as a PR guru – in fact she might've been better at being Lynne Franks than Lynne

Franks. I can see her now, bronze Birkenstocks tucked beneath a glass desk piled with the latest issue of *PR Week* and international editions of *Vogue*, black-and-white photographs of grateful celebrities on the wall behind her, on the phone to Harvey Weinstein about a *Save the Planet* concert, effortlessly persuading him to waive all his fees. But Lady Birkie wasn't in it for the money – she networked for the greater good of Norfolk and Suffolk because she was kind and generous, all the way from her coiffed auburn curls to the manicured toenails showcased by her bronze Birkies. She immediately started laying plans for literary lunches, introducing me to the managers of several local bookshops and organising my first-ever book reading.

I might not have considered *Yoga School Dropout*, a travel memoir describing my search for mystic Indians, Tantric bliss and a steady boyfriend in the yoga schools of India, a natural for the Southwold literary festival but Lady Birkie was very definite on the matter. She arranged for me to do my reading in the town's most glamorous clothes shop; Collen and Clare was overflowing with this season's most gorgeous must-haves and an expansive collection of Hunter wellingtons in every shade, from baby pink to silver. As I perched on a raspberry velvet sofa to do my reading I wondered if this would be the most elegant audience I would ever talk to – the ladies sipped from pretty bone china cups and saucers and nibbled on pink-and-blue iced cup cakes, this season's handbags at their pretty feet. After the reading the ladies shared their own experiences of ashram life and, in the case of one seventy-something grandmother, the details of her recent single-handed trek through the Himalayas. They kindly bought copies of my book as

David looked on proudly from in amongst the Hunter wellingtons display. I left with several pink-and-blue iced cupcakes in my pockets and a big Collen and Clare bag in my hand – it contained a must-have scarf wrapped in layers of gorgeous tissue paper – purchased with the day's profits.

By going only on personal recommendation we managed to avoid the worst of the 'NFN's. According to Keith Skipper, a commentator on Norfolk ways, the acronym was coined by A. N. Wilson in the *Sunday Telegraph* in 1991:

'I know of a medical practice in rural East Anglia where the majority of the patients are inbred, hare-lipped, mental defectives. When they put their boot faces round the surgery door and pour out their tales of woe to the doctor, the GP writes "NFN" on their notes. It means "Normal for Norfolk".'

We never came across any 'inbred, hare-lipped, mental defectives' but inevitably, despite our best efforts, we did encounter some 'Normal for Norfolk' behaviour. We wondered whether building a tower only to find it too heavy to put on the main building of the Beccles church may have been the earliest recorded example of 'NFN' behaviour, though technically speaking St Michael's was in Suffolk – perhaps they used Norfolk builders?

The most common latter-day 'NFN' practice we experienced was that of spending hours pricing up a job and not following through with a quote. Then there was the fridge repair guy who couldn't work out why water was collecting in the bottom of the fridge.

'It's a mystery, I've been repairing fridges for thirty years,' he said, staring at the stagnant pool of water.

As a fridge's basic function is temperature control I decided to hazard a guess. 'I don't know,' I said gently, 'do you think it might be because the bottom of the fridge is too warm?'

'Do you know,' he said, standing up and scratching his head, 'I think you might be right.'

Then there was the well-meaning policeman who parked his car under the tilting haystack as he directed traffic away from the scene.

Then there was the trip to a bathroom supplies shop with Tony the Tiler.

'You can't take that shower screen,' said the saleswoman indignantly as Tony picked it up to carry it to his van.

'Why not?' I asked.

'Because someone else has bought it.'

'Who's that?' I asked.

'Someone called Lucy Edge has bought it.'

'*I'm* Lucy Edge,' I said.

'No, you're not.'

'Yes, I am.'

The owner of the shop had to step in to verify that I was not an imposter hellbent on stealing Lucy Edge's shower screen. Tony told me it wasn't the first time the saleswoman had been a bit 'NFN'.

'You can't call yourself Tony the Tiler,' she told him the first time she'd seen his van.

'Why not?'

'Because there's already a Tony the Tiler.'

'That's me,' said Tony the Tiler.

'No, there's another Tony the Tiler.'

'No, there isn't. It's me, I'm Tony the Tiler.'

'No, there's another Tony the Tiler and he won't be very pleased if you pass yourself off as Tony the Tiler.'

In the end, to prevent the woman having a heart attack, Tony the Tiler had to agree that he wouldn't try to take any business away from Tony the Tiler.

Then there was the twenty-year-old Walter Mitty character that somehow persuaded himself he was a landscape gardener and tree surgeon capable of trimming five feet off forty trees single-handedly, and in three days, for a grand total of £225. Day one didn't go so well. He came to the back door a total of eight times in two hours – first to borrow a step ladder, then a chainsaw, then an extension lead, then a measuring tape, then to tell me he couldn't trim the front of the trees because his mate had just told him he might kill them, then to tell me his other mate had told him he couldn't cut down trees containing birds' nests, then to tell me he couldn't cut the second line of trees because they were on the other side of a two-foot-high fence, then to tell me he'd have to come back tomorrow with two lads to help him, and charge us £3,000. He didn't come back again.

5

'I didn't marry Trisha
for her tits'

Although we were beginning to meet local people, we hadn't yet met our tribe and spent a large part of the summer importing our friends. Gabriele, Andrea and Poppy came to celebrate my birthday in September. It was a gloriously hot weekend and we arranged ourselves on blankets in the garden, Andrea lying in the shade and entertaining us with stories from the front line of Internet dating, Poppy chasing the sun and wondering where to locate her boutique hotel, Gabriele chasing her children around the garden as they chased butterflies and the rotating water sprinkler, as I moved in between the blankets proffering birthday cake, iced lemonade and, a little later, Pimms. We used Gabriele's two children as an excuse to participate in the Beccles Duck Race – an annual event in which thousands of yellow rubber ducks are released from the confines of their bathtub, kitted out with headscarves, chef's hats, pink afros and the like and dropped into the river from a crane high above the town quay. We ran wild, blowing whistles in encouragement, but to no avail – our two ducks, dressed in miniature tweed caps reminiscent of David's own signature look, got lost somewhere between the start and finish line. We suspected sabotage but were unable to provide proof.

It was Poppy we saw most often. She called in every two or three weeks on her way back from a project she was doing in north Norfolk, renovating an old mill for a pop star. Both project and Poppy's love life were doing well – she'd split up with the younger man in favour of an older man, an architect and recently divorced Canadian with two grown-up children, soon to be affectionately nicknamed 'the Groover from Vancouver'. One weekend they donned their cowboy boots and hats and joined us for a Country and Western festival in the grounds of Strumpshaw Hall, a few miles north of Beccles. David was very excited; he'd always loved the Nashville sound and had recently discovered a country and western station on our brand-new Internet radio. Under something approaching constant exposure I was also becoming somewhat of an enthusiast. David had cowboy boots from the days he worked as a Saturday boy at R. Soles on the Kings Road but he didn't have a cowboy hat so I lent him a bright pink one I'd acquired along the way and, as it was a little big, he wore it balanced on his tweed cap – thus cleverly combining nods to both the country and the west.

We drove across the flatlands of east Norfolk, passing through villages consisting of a handful of houses and a barking dog, and took the car across the River Yare on the Reedham Ferry, the only way of getting from our house to the northern side of the Broads without driving more than thirty miles out of our way. There was a bit of a queue for the chain-pulled ferry as it only held three cars at a time so we patiently waited our turn, which gave us plenty of time to enjoy the sight of motorboats ploughing through the glassy water, and to wave at the end-of-season tourists enjoying a late afternoon drink outside the pretty white pub on the opposite bank.

Weaving our way along a succession of ever-more narrow lanes, overhanging trees creating dark tunnels through which rays of sunshine occasionally flashed, we eventually arrived at our destination. Behind the half-hidden gate a vast American flag fluttered, and beyond that lay a small village of Winnebagos. A draconian gate keeper insisted that we remain at the gate until the end of the afternoon set – no matter – we made our own entertainment, performing an unofficial line dance to the strains of John C. King's 'The Lord Made a Hobo out of Me' while the dragon stood at the gate breathing smoke and fire. We got chatting to the proud owner of a silver Airstream trailer parked at the gate, he offered us a beer and a tour of the interior. I'm not sure that its velour-covered furniture and sheepskin rugs scored any points with Poppy but it was almost the size of my old flat and had every human comfort – a double bed and a shower cubicle, a kitchen with plenty of work surfaces, an L-shaped sofa and a driving seat that doubled as an armchair.

When we were finally allowed in it was immediately apparent that Strumpy was a different kind of festival. For a start the loos were the cleanest I have seen anywhere – the last festival I'd been to had used tactical advertising to great effect on the back of the loo doors – *Don't Look Down* was the title of a new single by the Guillemots and the best advice the organisers of Latitude could've given anyone using the toilets. Here at Strumpy, as the Groover from Vancouver said, planting his thumbs into his waistcoat pocket and rocking on his heels, not only could you look down with confidence, 'You sure could eat off one of those.' They were also the highest loos I have ever seen – perhaps to help out those with mobility issues. You see Strumpy had the oldest festival attendees ever; we watched as determined women in motorised wheelchairs put their hand on the accelerator to get to the front of the food queue and a gang of seventy-year-old ladies wearing red, blue and green satin saloon dresses with plunging black lace necklines walked hand in hand with greying Davy Crocketts, whiskered Confederates and portly Red Indians.

Poppy braved the wrath of the Red Indians to take their photograph and I wondered if the Groover might be creating north-west London's first log cabin next year – there between the Regency terraces overlooking Regent's Park would nestle a pioneer home with double doors opening onto handcrafted red cedar fireplaces, barn wood floors and wagon-wheel furniture, styled up with Navajo blankets, chandeliers made of elk antlers (naturally shed of course) and Leonard Reedy, 'Chicago's Cowboy Painter', oils. Poppy would organise the *Architectural Digest* photoshoots wearing a Native American headdress, vintage sterling silver concho belt and Indian green squash blossom necklace – more or less what she was wearing today.

The festival goers were also rather larger than average in size – this seemed to be in part explained by the limited food options: fish and chips or hamburgers and chips. Where was the fair trade Veggie Kitchen? Where was Captain Cobb, last seen at Latitude dispensing organic corn dripping with butter and chives? Where was Goodness Gracious and its vegetarian curries? Where was the organic falafel stand? And what was with the completely non biodegradable packaging? Where were the recycling bins? It had to be the least environmentally friendly event I had ever been to; clearly the remains of this festival would be with us a lot longer than its participants.

Entering the marquee it was clear that Strumpy occupied an alternative universe. It was the first music festival I'd ever been to that had chairs right up to the stage; behind the chairs were rows of tables on which family territories were marked out by piles of sweets and crisps. To either side of the chairs were two dance floors, one labelled 'Freestyle' and the other 'Line Dancing and Partners'. We watched the line dancers with awestruck wonder – they were executing the moves perfectly but curbing both their energy and enthusiasm; as the Groover from Vancouver said, 'are they dead, or asleep?'

That wasn't the only surprising thing about the dance floor – its borders demarcated the most inclusive place in the world – a person of seven could dance alongside a person of ninety and be part of the same flow, a fat person could dance alongside a thin person and not feel the difference, a person could be completely alone and still find themselves part of something, a person could come up, dance to half a song and go sit down again if they got bored, or tired of curbing their enthusiasm. By the time the band played a song in which Sheila was invited to pour another Tequila and take off her satin dress, we were all failing to curb our enthusiasm; David whirling me around and around in his tweed and pink hats, the only ethnic minority – apart from the Red Indians – for miles, the Groover expertly leading Poppy around the Freestyle dance floor with a precision that could've merited them a place on *Strictly Strumpy*. In the end we had to work hard to prise ourselves away – if they could only improve their food options and develop a little environmental awareness Strumpy would be a fine blueprint for all festivals.

Would we have to keep on importing our friends for ever? For a time I was worried whether we would be absorbed by the locals. Norfolk is traditionally suspicious of blow-ins, not surprising really considering that the early blow-ins, the Vikings, had raped, pillaged and set the churches on fire. There is a famous Norfolk saying, 'Progress is fine, as long as it doesn't change anything', and so far the Up From London second-homers in search of art galleries, boutique hotels, Michelin-starred restaurants and designer clothes shops had concentrated themselves in Burnham Market, leaving most of the county, especially the east, to the Norfolk born and bred.

I'd grown up sixty miles away in a small village just outside Saffron Walden in Essex, so at least my blow-in had been fairly short distance, though the twenty years I'd spent in London hadn't done me any favours in the locals' eyes, but David, well, he was the subject of substantial continental drift. What were they making of him, 'the first Paki in the village'? Beccles wasn't known for its ethnic diversity – I'd spotted a Vietnamese woman in Tesco and we'd seen a Rasta on one of the floats at the carnival back in July – but generally the county had a white hue last seen in London around 1800.

I wasn't too worried about our prospects – David had a lot of practice at blowing in – he was born in Karachi to Indian parents and had spent a happy childhood playing cricket and running kites through the city streets, but the family had to leave Pakistan when Bhutto put a death threat on his father, a fearless investigative journalist, for breaking news of the slayings in what would become Bangladesh.

Yvonne, David's mother, flew to her brother's house in Rome with two suitcases and five children before journeying to London a few days later. His father travelled separately to ensure the family's safety, via Afghanistan and Iran. The then editor of the *Sunday Times*, Harold Evans, devoted the 13 June 1971 front page to Anthony Mascarenhas's story; the headline read 'Genocide!' The book of the story, *Bangladesh: a Legacy of Blood*, was dedicated to 'Yvonne and our children – who have also paid the price.' The twelve-year-old David made an initially difficult transition, wandering the deserted streets of Ladbroke Grove, wondering where all the other cricket-playing, kite-running children were, but in the end he settled, dumbing down so he wouldn't be teased for being so far ahead in his lessons, and moderating his perfect vowels to fit in with the other children at his Roman Catholic school. Finding his place in Norfolk? Well surely that would be a walk in the park.

Finally, one September Sunday, we got our lucky break. We'd just emptied our fridge of Lukullus Juniper sausages, U Jedrusia dumplings and yogurt, when we received an invitation to Sunday lunch hosted by networker extraordinaire Lady Birkie, and her husband.

Two weeks later, on the last hot day of the year, we drove to the other side of Beccles, down a lavender-lined drive – a drive so long that despite the fact we passed through the electronic gates on time we were actually ten minutes late when we finally arrived at the front door of the impressive stone manor house. We stood nervously in front of a statue of a prancing lion, clutching a bottle of wine.

A woman who might best be described as a maid opened the door and we were immediately engulfed in the affections of two lithe rusty gold-coloured dogs that she informed us were Lord Birkie's Hungarian Vizslas; thus accompanied we were shown straight through to the back of the house where ten guests were already assembled on a stone terrace overlooking a vast expanse of tropical plants, walled enclosures and greenhouses that shimmered in the heat of a fierce sun.

'How many acres do you have here?' I asked Lord Birkie, gratefully sipping the large glass of Pimms that he thrust into my hand as I drank in his chiselled features – he must have been sixty but he had the broad shoulders and strong arms of a man half his age.

'About five hundred,' he replied gruffly, turning several sizzling supersized steaks on a state-of-the-art barbecue. 'I don't like neighbours.'

'Is the beef local?' I asked, relieved that there wasn't a Lukullus Juniper sausage in sight.

'Yes, we have our own herd,' he replied, kicking away the Vizslas and pouring himself another drink. I noticed his Pimms had been substituted for whisky, which he was drinking neat.

'You seem to be quite an expert at barbecuing,' I said, polishing off my Pimms (it was hot) and surreptitiously removing an alcohol-soaked strawberry that had dropped unbidden into my cleavage.

'Learned the art in Argentina when I was playing polo,' he said, running his fingers through the flop of hair that threatened his sight, 'ate it pretty well raw over there. If I had it my way I'd just wipe its arse and bring it to the table,' he sighed, 'but people here seem to like it a little more well done.'

By the time I joined the other guests I was feeling distinctly, what Lord Birkie might've described as 'squiffy'.

They were all mildly pissed when we'd arrived, and remarkably, despite the heat of the afternoon, their state of inebriation remained seemingly unchanged. Where did they put it all?

I have subsequently found this to be a bit of a theme – whereas Londoners will stumble out of bars and vomit all over the pavement, the natives of Norfolk would consider it seriously impolite to appear in the slightest bit affected by drinking three bottles of red in one sitting. When Walpole called them 'roast beefs fashioned in human form' he wasn't being entirely flattering but was there a back-handed compliment in there too? Was he not, at least in part, referring to a certain sturdiness of constitution?

Perhaps the secret also lies in the quality of the alcohol consumed – whereas a Londoner might endeavour to place an unwanted bottle of screw-top Chardonnay at a party, believing a quick unseen deposit on the kitchen worktop to be a suitable dumping ground, there is no such anonymity in Norfolk – the host is always aware of the quality of his guest's contribution, and will in all likelihood take it as an indicator of the quality of his guest. Anyway I was glad we'd taken something decent – I just wish we'd taken more of it.

Lady Birkie whisked David away and I stood, not really listening to a conversation about the rising cost of stable girls, as I took in the unspoken dress code – which we seemed to have got wrong. David had come wearing George Michael's denim blouson, recalling the 1983 *Club Tropicana* video, when he should have been in mustard or red cotton trousers and jacket. I was in a Cacharel graphic print low-cut top, slouchy flares and my white wedges, and should have worn a large sun hat, tailored cream linen suit and immaculate scarlet nails like our hostess. Oh well, there was nothing I could do about it now. I tried hanging on the timeless skirts of Dom Antony but he was deeply engrossed in a conversation about cricket so I ended up with a Sex Therapist.

An attractive and stylish brunette in her late forties, she carried off a ruby red figure-hugging shift dress rather better than most women of twenty, despite having had several children. She must've been hit on a lot when she was an air hostess but sadly for me she'd learned the art of discretion early on. We chatted for a while about the joys of three-day stopovers and flying the friendly skies back in the eighties, the appeal of a career as a Sex Therapist (working from home, relationship building, using her brain), and the use of cling film in the sexual act.

'It's much more common than you might think,' she said authoritatively.

David joined us while I was doing mental gymnastics trying to work out how cling film might be used in sex.

She looked us up and down.

David and I looked at each other.

She paused a moment.

'You two still have "It",' she pronounced.

Ah well, it was comforting to know that even though we weren't producing children we were still hot.

Lady Birkie swooped down and moved me swiftly on, introducing me to a sparrow-like creature of the minutest proportions; I started, and finished, by asking her how she kept her figure – did it involve a strict diet?

'I eat three Mars bars a day,' she confided.

'Nothing else?' I asked.

'No, I ride horses all day and that's what keeps me going.'

I wasn't sure if she was joking or not but it sounded like my kind of diet; probably not on the recommended list of fertility foods though.

Lady Birkie kept me circulating, this time introducing me to a whiskery ex-guardsman. We soon got on to the subject of moving.

'Oh, it can be quite a thing,' he said, sympathetically. 'Who moved you?'

'A man I found in the Yellow Pages,' I informed him. 'I couldn't believe how much stuff I had – fifty-six boxes you know – but I saved myself more than a hundred pounds by using old crisp boxes from Waitrose.'

The gentleman persevered, still looking for common ground. Something told me wooden tea chests hand-packed by overalled men in white gloves had been closer to his experience.

He soldiered on. 'Are you reaching the end of your unpacking?' he enquired politely. 'Have you hung your pictures yet?'

I momentarily toyed with the idea of claiming that I just didn't know where to put all my old masters but I'm afraid that I rather let myself and my hostess down by admitting that I didn't have any.

Was David faring any better? A red-faced Irishman had taken him aside and was breathing heavily into his ear, 'Don't worry about not fitting in, old chap, I've been here years and I never have. I don't let it bother me, though.' I'm not sure he'd taken his own advice – I heard him later telling everyone that 'Of course, all my children went to Eton and Oxford' as he knocked back another whisky.

We sat down to eat. The steaks were the biggest I have ever seen, as were the glasses of red wine that replaced our Pimms. Our host poured himself another whisky and took his place at the head of the table. The man sitting to my right, a local landowner in mustard-coloured cotton trousers and jacket, was keen to establish common ground.

'Do you have dogs?'

'No, but I'd love a chocolate brown Labrador,' I gushed, grateful not to have to answer the usual question about children.

'That shows how little you know about dogs,' said the landowner, laughing. 'You see chocolate brown Labs are stupid dogs, they're only bred for their colour, and the best dogs are bred for their intelligence. That's what you are looking for – an intelligent dog...'

'I like Lord Birkie's dog,' I interrupted, 'how about a Hungarian Vizsla?'

'They're great hunting dogs but a Terrier would be the best choice for a house dog,' he said, closing down the debate with some expertise. 'Now, what are you doing with your stables?'

I found it disconcerting that other people knew our house so well and was reluctant to share our plans. 'Um... not sure yet... we aren't very horsy...' I stammered. I was beginning to feel as I did when I first went to Mysore and everyone was called Rainbow or River and had practised yoga in their mother's womb; I was never going to fit in. I managed to choke back the next sentence – in which I would've announced our intention to convert them into a yoga studio for weekend workshops. Somehow I thought it might've been a conversation stopper.

'They were built in the seventies,' explained the landowner. 'One of your predecessors had them put up – she was mad about horses, used to ride them into Beccles and tie them up at Barclays bank or the traffic lights.'

I'd also heard that she rode in the woods at two in the morning with a torch attached to her stirrup and that she liked to wander naked round the garden but I decided not to mention either snippet. You never knew where people stood on these matters.

The large lady sitting opposite me introduced herself by talking a great deal about her huge bosoms, in fact she called them her 'puppies' (if they were puppies I can only begin to imagine what the fully grown versions would look like – had Norfolk grown its very own naturally blessed Jordan?). She spent quite a lot of the lunch telling them off for misbehaving in the heat. There was talk of 'warm rivulets' and 'panting'. This warmed up the men beside her who felt permission had been granted to compare all the bosoms at the table; the red-trousered man sitting to my left peered down my low-cut top and pronounced me 'not big in that department'.

And I was wearing my cleavage-boosting bra.

'Ah well, never mind,' he continued jollily, 'I didn't marry Trisha for her tits.'

I suppressed the urge to retaliate with 'and I don't expect Trisha married you for your dick' by downing the rest of my glass in one. I found out later I would probably have been wrong on that count – his nicknames were 'King Pin' and 'Strong Prong'.

It was around that point that I caught up with everyone else's state of inebriation and the rest of the afternoon passed in a hazy blur.

*

It was hard to recall many of the specifics of that lunch but one of the few things that stuck in my mind was a conversation about Great Yarmouth. Everyone had been very down on it, describing it as 'chavvy' and 'not our kind of place'. I looked it up in my book *Literary Norfolk*; the town had enjoyed heady days as the herring capital of the world – to Dickens's David Copperfield it had smelled of fish, pitch, oakum and tar. To Daniel Defoe, visiting Yarmouth in 1722, it had the 'finest quay in England if not in Europe' with merchants' houses 'like palaces rather than the dwelling houses of private men'. By the time Henry James arrived, in the early years of the twentieth century, something fundamental had shifted and he wrote that 'miles of cockneyfied seafront… now strikes the wrong note so continuously that I, for my part, become conscious, on the spot, of a chill to the spirit of research.'

Feeling lonely after David's departure one Monday I decided to satisfy my curiosity and spend the afternoon there. I was determined to have an authentic seaside experience, starting with some fish and chips – I have to say I struggled a bit to find the fish and chip shop of my dreams and ended up asking for a recommendation in a bed and breakfast with flock wallpaper and an indoor fountain – this being early October the only inhabitants were the gnomes who lived in a grotto, who were enjoying a perpetual summer lit by orange and red fairy lights. The landlady suggested I try the Winter Gardens – a giant greenhouse purchased by the Great Yarmouth Corporation in 1904 to improve Wellington Pier. I settled down with my plate of chips and read about Jordan and Peter Andre's latest escapades in a tatty gossip magazine while listening to the excited screams of children hurtling down the giant slides in the 'wild adventure park' at the opposite end of the indoor garden.

I felt so cosy and warm, so centrally heated by my chips, that I hardly felt the icy wind cutting in across the mile of sandy beach as I walked up to Britannia Pier – the sea like dirty coffee stirred up in a sudsy washing-up bowl. From the beach I could see twenty or more wind turbines rising out of the distant sea like H. G. Wells's Martian War Tripods – although there was no sign of their Death Rays or Black Smoke in the chalky sky. I watched the fishermen casting off the last line of the day – their spikes so large that getting hooked and used as human bait seemed a real possibility. The smell of candy floss, ice cream and penny sweets drifted towards the beach from the cafés and kiosks lining the Golden Mile – taking the bite out of the salty air. Endless arcades lined the other side of the road where there was a different kind of fishing going on – the kind where you pay a pound to watch a claw on the end of a miniature crane pick up a pink teddy bear, and then drop it – did I chance a pound? No, I'd suffered enough psychological damage as a child at the Morecambe Pleasure Beach not to want to go there again.

I arrived at the top of Yarmouth's Golden Mile to find a queue forming for a dance show about to start on Britannia Pier. Why not? I didn't have anything else to do and it might be quite good – there were ads for forthcoming shows from local Jim Davidson, the Four Tops and Elkie 'Pearl's a Singer' Brooks. Even Elvis would be coming back from the grave for a night at the pier. I stood in line and slowly made my way past 650 feet of temptation – the toffee apple, doughnut and waffle stands smelled so deliciously sweet they made my tummy rumble despite the large quantity of chips I'd just consumed. I read a tourist leaflet that informed me that the pier was lucky to be in one piece – it fell victim to a renegade schooner just a year after it was built in 1854 – and over the next hundred years it burned to the ground four more times, although ironically it withstood the war when the Germans dropped more than 8,000 bombs on Great Yarmouth.

The show, put on by one of the big dance schools in the area, was a sellout and I sat with all the proud mums as children who'd surely only taken their first steps the month before, ran around the stage as twinkling stars. Each dance featured children another year older – from twinkling two-year-olds to five-year-old forest bugs to ten-year-old trees to slender eighteen-year-old running streams in shimmering metallic grey leotards. I felt a twinge at the sight of these children on the stage, and at the proud young mums in the audience, all so much younger than me. The show reached a crescendo two hours later when thirty mums in identical pink cowboy hats and tap shoes whooped and hollered their way through a faultless performance that would have breathed new life into the *Strictly Strumpy* line dancing competition.

Walking back to my car I passed a fully grown man riding his daughter's pink Barbie scooter as she searched busily for sea shells – that for me was Great Yarmouth at its best; it wasn't going to win any style awards any time soon, but I liked the playful spirit of the place – it was uncomplicated fun for children and a place for an adult to let go – to wear a star-spangled cowboy hat and kick up high. I thought of David and his tweed and pink hats and looked forward to the day we'd ride our children's scooters.

6

'Stay behind the yellow socks'

The bad news was that I hadn't yet found my tribe. The good news was that, just over three months after I left London, my internal clock was beginning to adjust to Norfolk Mean Time and I found myself no longer 'living a short distance from my body'. I began to enjoy mardling, and I stopped feeling guilty about doing nothing. In fact I rather embraced it – I'd go for a walk in the woods, kicking up the yellow leaves that fell in a continuous shower from the ash, maple and sycamore trees, watching squirrels climbing towards the autumn sun that filtered weakly through the branches. I'd admire the red of the rosehips that popped out of the hedges, often feeling that I was being watched by hundreds of pairs of eyes – field mice, voles, pheasants, wood pigeon, hares; sometimes we would surprise each other and a hare or partridge would shoot out of the field into the distance. I'd return with my pockets stuffed with raspberries and blackberries that I'd picked from the thorny hedgerows. Back in our sitting room I'd sit by the window and watch 'old hush-wing' silently cruising in the twilight, returning to its nest in the barn beside our house.

David walked with me on weekends, picking up fallen

apples and pears to give to the horses at the local rescue centre – an exercise that initially petrified us – all those teeth and all that slobber – but soon became a favourite pastime. The more we explored the more we came to appreciate just how much work goes into conserving the land; cycling the lanes bordering the local farms we'd see fields rich with oil-seed rape, barley, sugar beet or maize divided by squarely trimmed hedgerows, the ditches scooped out, clean and empty of weeds, and the farm buildings as neat and tidy as the rows of pensioners' bungalows that lined the outskirts of Beccles.

One of my favourite walks was from the old bridge on the outskirts of Beccles towards the Geldeston Locks Inn, marking the end of the navigable waters on the River Waveney. It was hard to imagine that this freshwater river, home to otters, kingfishers and marsh harriers, had once been a saltwater estuary of the sea. Hundreds of years ago the estuary had been so rich in herrings that the Abbot of Edmundsbury had to pay 30,000 of them in tax – I don't know what the rate of taxation was back in the years of the Domesday Book but I would think it safe to assume that he would still have been left with hundreds of thousands for his own consumption.

I'd admire the pretty riverfront houses sloping down to the river's edge on my left, some were modern, some were old, and they all had lawns that, even in October, looked as green and soft as just-thrown-down rugs. I'd try to imagine life in nineteenth-century Beccles – looking in between these houses I could see the narrow scores, the lanes going down to the river, where the wherries would've discharged wheat, coal and barley, a trade that ended when the railway arrived in 1854. Now the river traded in tourists – it was home to several holiday hire boat companies, the duck race and the

Beccles sailing regatta, which had been held most summers for the past two hundred years.

Eventually the houses petered out, making way for a boatyard and the 'new' open air swimming pool, a local fixture since the 1880s. The place must've seen some changing fashions; I wished I'd been a witness to the 1930s customer who enjoyed parading up and down clad only in a bowler hat and towel. After the pool came the boathouse and garden plots, some of which sported carefully tended lawns and little houses with gingham curtains. I imagined myself sunbathing in a deck chair, contemplating an afternoon on my boat – a motor cruiser I'd call 'The Cappuccino Guru'. I'd relax on ancient faded-out cushions, eating strawberries and sipping Pimms with Poppy, Andrea and Gabriele, a white-capped David in a windcheater, deck shoes and pressed cotton shorts at the helm.

We first met the Sheriff emerging from the local woods on his green Kawasaki Mole. He had several large tubs of seed in the back of the truck and a determined look on his face. He slowed to a halt and we introduced ourselves. He explained that he was the gamekeeper for one of the local landowners and was having trouble with his pheasants who, despite his best efforts to keep them contained with regular feeding, kept wandering off.

'The shooting season starts next week and the numbers are about ten per cent down this year,' he said with concern, carefully flattening his white hair to his head. 'They seem to have migrated and I don't know where they've gone.'

'I think they're all at our place,' I ventured. 'You should see them – they make a funny sight – the partridges walk in single file, nine or ten of them in a line, the tallest at the front, the smallest at the back, the rabbits zigzagging playfully in between them. The pheasants sit in a row on top of our stables, puffing up their chests and looking down on the chaos below.'

The Sheriff tried his best to look amused but was clearly upset that the birds he'd worked so hard to rear had taken early retirement in our garden.

The following week he arrived at the back door looking mighty relieved. The first shoot of the season had been a big success and, as if to prove it, he produced a rabbit out of his Driza Bone hat. 'It's a young doe – should be very tender – just soak it in salt for a couple of hours first,' he told me. 'And here's some pigeon for you.'

He saw my face.

'Don't worry – it's nothing to be afraid of. It tastes like dark chicken and is great in a curry.'

The Sheriff responded enthusiastically to the offer of a cup of tea and took up position at the head of the kitchen table, filling out the carver and nobly turning down a slice of cake.

'I'm a type two diabetic and I had a blood sugar count of twenty-seven last weekend.'

'What should it be?'

'Oh, between five and seven,' he chuckled, his cheeks reddening, his blue eyes glinting. 'We had a family party and I don't know what happened – I just went a bit mad.'

I put the cake away.

'So, young lady,' he said, 'do you want to come on the next shoot? I've asked the Squire and he says that you're very welcome.'

The Squire was the Sheriff's employer, landlord and the owner of a substantial estate up the road.

'I don't know,' I said uncertainly. 'I've never shot before; I am not sure how good I'd be.'

'Oh, don't worry about that,' he said, laughing. 'Women can't shoot. You'd be beating.'

'Beating?'

'A beater beats the birds out of the bushes. They tend to hide in the brambles so your job is to get them to fly up and out into the paths of the guns.'

The Sheriff explained that the Squire ran nine or ten shoots a year with an average of seven so-called 'Guns', that is, guns with men attached to them. The Guns were local landowners or wealthy businessmen. The Squire wasn't in it to make money – he wanted to provide sport for his friends but the idea was to reciprocate shoot days, either on their land or, if they didn't have any, to buy days from commercial enterprises who charged anything from twenty to twenty-five pounds a bird.

'And how many do they shoot in a day?' I asked.

'Oh,' said the Sheriff rocking back in his seat, 'they can shoot between 100 and 500 per day – it can get rather expensive if they're a good shot.'

Five hundred birds in a day? That wasn't a shoot, that was a massacre.

'Isn't it dangerous?' I asked weakly, 'especially if they aren't good shots?'

'Oh yes,' said the Sheriff solemnly, 'it's a very dangerous sport. Have you got a broom?'

I didn't have a broom to hand so I gave him a mop. I didn't ask why; he'd been a copper for thirty-two years before he was a gamekeeper and there was something in his manner that didn't encourage you to ask questions.

'An experienced Gun will hold the gun aloft like so,' he said, standing his full six feet and pointing the head of the mop at the ceiling. 'An inexperienced Gun will hold the gun at waist height like so,' he said, demonstrating the position with the mop at ninety degrees to his substantial girth. I could see why that might be a problem. 'Never forget that a loaded gun is a lethal weapon,' he said, his blue eyes glinting.

He must have seen my alarm. 'Don't worry,' he assured me, 'we haven't had many deaths. Someone lost an eye once but they got a bungalow out of it; that's the going rate, a bungalow for an eye.'

Was he joking? I was seriously wondering if this was a good idea.

'You know that pheasants wouldn't exist if it wasn't for shooting,' explained the Sheriff. 'We only shoot the males and this enables us to manage the population – cock pheasants like a harem of five or six females – successful breeding maintains a ratio of twenty per cent male to eighty per cent female. The feed we leave supports the smaller birds too. We use the fields to grow cover crops like maize to provide the living space for the pheasants – we would make more money if we grew wheat, but it's not about that. We are preserving the countryside – as well as pheasants and woodcock we might kill some ducks to maintain the breeding ratios – if three or four males try to mate with the female at the same time they can end up killing her. Partridges aren't very successful breeders so we shoot both sexes and restock. We will also kill vermin if we find any – magpies, jays, crows, grey squirrels.'

We moved on to practicalities.

I was advised to bring a packed lunch and hope for some soup.

'What shall I wear?' I asked.

'A denim miniskirt?' quipped the Sheriff.

We settled on a waterproof hat, Barbour, jeans and wellies.

By the time I reached the end of the long drive I was feeling distinctly nervous – especially when I saw a knot of people dressed in plus fours. They looked so smart – Barbours and peaked tweed caps were coordinated with German smooth-haired Pointers, Hungarian Vizslas and yellow Labradors. It struck me that the British do country style better than anyone else in the world – they look so good that even the Italians copy it, buying up Barbours and Hunters with an enthusiasm usually reserved for their football teams. I thought it a shame that this wasn't our national dress – Barbours and plus fours would look a heck of a lot better than the three-quarter trousers and tank tops proudly sported by the nation at airports and shopping malls. But in the style stakes the Sheriff was in a class of his own – he wore a Driza-Bone hat, freshly laundered white shirt, a brown tweed waistcoat, matching plus fours, yellow socks, and a yellow tie covered in teddy bears.

As this wasn't a look I could easily emulate I selected the driver of the shoot wagon as my style guru for the day – she wore jeans and Hunters with just the right amount of mud spattered upon them, a brown Driza-Bone mac and matching hat. She was mad about horses, and before I even knew her name I'd been enrolled as a judge at a forthcoming horse show.

'But I don't know anything about horses,' I protested.

'Oh, don't worry about that, dear,' she said, 'it's fool-proof.'

We stood in a circle and introduced ourselves. Before I got a chance to open my mouth the Sheriff had done my work for me and told everyone that I was from London. Everyone smiled politely but I could tell that in some small way the power had shifted away from me. I dug my hands deep into the pockets of my Barbour and contemplated my shiny new Hunters – I wished that I'd sprayed them with some mud before I left the house, and I probably hadn't helped my case by wearing a sparkly blue hat with ear flaps and a bobble.

Each beater took an orange flag. They were all rolled up and I inadvertently took the Keeper's flag – this turned out to be something of a sin. 'The only sin worse would be to shoot a hen,' said the Sheriff sternly as he slowly unrolled the flag and with a final theatrical flourish revealed the word '**BANG!**' written in felt tip pen across the centre.

'The forfeit is to kiss the Keeper,' quipped one of the beaters.

'I had to kiss one of the beaters last year,' admitted the Sheriff, 'but I didn't like his aftershave.'

I managed to get on the wagon without any further incident, shoving my handbag packed with make-up, loo paper and some sticky ginger cake that I'd bought from the local farmers' market under the bench. We bounced around on the benches – some of us clinging more securely to our place than others. Size helped to root a person, as did the tightness of the packing – passengers on a Central Line Tube in the rush hour had more room than we did. There was a lot of banter about sitting on knees, most of it aimed at the four women on the wagon – two of whom were in full commando gear, and the third of whom had a Rottweiler. Personally I wouldn't have messed with them.

I noticed that the buttocks of the German Pointer sitting opposite me were quivering.

'What's going on with your dog?' I asked his owner.

'Nerves,' he confessed, 'her buttocks look like my stomach feels.'

He did look rather pale. I asked him what he was worried about.

'Will I shoot anything? Will my dog stay under control?' He swallowed hard.

Suddenly waving a flag around and staying out of the way of stray bullets didn't seem to be such a big challenge.

We tumbled out into the middle of a field; there were no familiar landmarks and the wagon had no windows so I had absolutely no idea where I was.

The Sheriff had explained that there would be seven 'drives' across different fields so each man would get several turns to shoot. My instructions were simple; all I had to do was walk across the field shooting my flag so it screamed **'BANG!'**

'You have to whip it so it sounds like a gun,' the Sheriff informed me. 'Crack it down really hard.'

He gathered the beaters around him like a coach at half-time. 'We want all the birds flying up in the same direction so the Guns can get a clear look at them,' instructed the Sheriff. 'Fan out in a line, marking yourself against your neighbour.'

I must've looked worried.

'Just keep behind me; stay behind the yellow socks and you won't go wrong.'

It sounded simple but somehow we managed to get into quite a mess. We were an unruly lot.

'Stay behind the yellow socks!' shouted the Sheriff, blowing hard on his police issue whistle – a relic from his days as a copper. His face turned a dark shade of red. I lost track of the number of times he told us, and so evidently did Pubic, a wiry, short, curly black-haired Terrier, who clearly didn't like to follow instructions, running so fast after hares that its little legs appeared not to touch the ground.

'She's that quick she does half an hour in twenty minutes,' said Des her owner. 'She's much faster than my last dog – even though it was a dash-hound.'

The Rottweiler turned out to be scared of shot and ran away, in the direction of one of the faraway Guns. He was returned, tail between his legs, to the wagon and from there he was sent home to Great Yarmouth in disgrace.

I wasn't a natural at flag waving but eventually I got into a rhythm – pretending I was in a yoga class and making figures of eight with my flag in time with my breath. Some of the beaters made noises – 'Hey hey,' coaxed the Sheriff, others rolled their tongues, I thought about chanting '*Om*', but somehow using the symbol designed to blot out thoughts and thus increase oneness with the universe didn't seem appropriate. I settled for copying the Sheriff.

I was beginning to enjoy the day – the camaraderie, the banter, the enthusiasm of the dogs scenting the air, the crunch of woodland under foot, the rhythmic cracking of flags, and the landscape lying flat as an oil painting. I'd almost forgotten why I was there – it felt like a day out in the country with new friends. So seeing the first bird falling out of the sky was a shock. There it was soaring upwards, its red, blue, brown and gold plumage sharpened against the deep blue sky, and suddenly '**BANG!**' it was spiralling head first towards the ground. Occasionally the bird stuttered in mid-flight, tried to rise, then lost the battle and careered into a wood. Two birds were so spooked they garrotted themselves on electricity pylons, and one bird seemed to simply die of fright. They were picked up by the dogs and carried back to the Gun who took them to the game wagon. The sight of the still-warm birds, so soft, so broken, piled one on top of the other hit me like a punch to the stomach.

I tried to pull myself together, reminding myself that these were birds that owed their lives to the shoot – and how was this any different to the cultivation of cattle and sheep for meat? As a carnivore I was sending animals to their death every day of the year. I reasoned that it was good for me to witness the killing first-hand – it would make me more appreciative of what was put on my plate. But that line of reasoning didn't really work, so when I saw a line of Guns with only one or two birds at the end of a drive I couldn't help but feel a little stab of joy. I must confess that I may at this point have begun to put a little less effort into ripping my flag through the air – and when the Sheriff asked me to guard the tracks leading out of the woods I may not have paid too much attention as the odd pheasant crossed to the other side.

The drives continued, each one quite different in character – through woods, across open fields, over a disused gravel pit where a bird was shot but lost. A golden Labrador was sent after it, following its master's whistle and vocal commands. It returned with quarry between its teeth – I was impressed until it got up close and we discovered it was holding a long-dead rabbit. I survived the Sheriff's constant banter:

'Is your hat keeping you warm, Lucy?'

'Do you need a rest, Lucy?'

'Is it all a bit much for our Londoner?'

'Can you beat the pheasant sitting on that wall?'

I remained amenable to the last, perhaps a little too amenable. It wasn't until I got within ten metres that I realised the pheasant on the wall was a wooden sculpture.

We stopped for elevenses – a plastic beaker of port and a McVities chocolate digestive. I tried not to worry that the Guns were also drinking, and that one of them only had one eye; he told me that he'd lost the other to a rogue nail – at least it wasn't a rogue bullet. I chatted with my fellow beaters and found, amongst others, a herbalist, a landscape gardener, a horse breeder, a Reiki healer, a technical marketer for JCB and the father of the detective superintendent who'd caught the Suffolk Strangler.

Actually there were a number of policemen on the shoot – perhaps it was because the Sheriff had worked in Lowestoft for a few years. He told me that when he'd moved from the London Belgravia beat, the biggest contrast, and the issue which gave him regular problems, was having to arrest people he knew; he used to have regular cups of tea with the station master on his Lowestoft beat and they became friends, then he had to arrest the station master's son for nicking a bicycle from the station platform – in full view of its owner. Apparently the work of today's police was a little less like a storyline from a Hovis ad.

'Lowestoft is bad for burglary and drugs, but not as bad as Yarmouth which is the brown capital of the East,' explained one of the policemen.

'"Brown" – do you mean hash?' I asked, thinking myself quite knowledgeable on these matters.

'Heroin,' said the policeman, giving me a sharp look.

Two hours later we stopped for lunch. We ate at the crossroads in the woods, the food cooked on a gas-fired stove. Des the plumber, owner of Pubic, had won a thirty-pound bet with the Sheriff and generously donated it to providing our lunch, hot dogs with brown sauce or tomato ketchup, minestrone soup and malt loaf with lashings of butter. I was very grateful to eat something hot – it'd been an hour since I last felt my toes and food had never tasted so good. As I stood thawing out I listened to Des who turned out to be the lunchtime entertainment.

On his plans to stay out late:

'As lads we always used to say, "if you're not in bed by half past nine you might as well go home".'

On the man who told me he 'didn't marry Trisha for her tits':

'Don't worry about it. Old King Pin told me that his dog had more pedigree than me.'

'Do you know how Des got that black eye?' asked the Sheriff, winking at me.

'He told me that he put a guinea fowl in the chicken shed and one of the chickens flew into his eye in a panic.'

'A likely tale,' said the Sheriff, chuckling, 'it was his wife of course – she wasn't getting what she wanted so "whack!"'

I looked at Des. I looked at the Sheriff. They were both beaming from ear to ear. An angry chicken or an angry wife? God knows where the truth lay.

After another three drives I was flagging – especially when I got stuck in some brambles and tore my jeans, much to the amusement of the Sheriff. Fortunately further sustenance came in the form of a tin of Celebrations chocolates, a bottle of whisky and the ginger cake that I'd bought. Strictly speaking I wasn't supposed to be drinking – Fertility Goddesses don't knock whisky back at four in the afternoon – but I was in danger of losing my toes to frostbite so it was purely medicinal. And it would've been rude not to – as the Squire put it, 'this is a shoot not a Methodist prayer meeting'. I poured a good measure of Teachers into my thermos flask of coffee and knocked it back.

On the last drive the Sheriff was a man on a mission. 'There are 400 birds in this field and I want to kill 100 of them,' he declared, but even his killer instincts couldn't dent the rosy glow that now surrounded me – ah – the cold air, the flap of flags, the setting sun. Only my toes remained inured to the effects of the thermos flask.

At the other end of the field we met the Squire, flushed with success. He posed for a photo with his prize – a brace of hard-to-shoot woodcock – and as we bumped around in the wagon on our way back to the farm, he spoke about other people's opposition to the sport.

'Why shouldn't we hunt and shoot? I find it wrong that some people should impose their views on others – it's still a free country, just about. We are preserving the countryside, and our traditions.'

He told me that he began shooting at the age of eight and shot his first bird at ten. 'I love it,' he said, 'it brings you closer to the land, and I like the party,' he added ruefully, adjusting his brown tweed cap, looking down at his large hands spread out across his plus fours, 'a little too much perhaps.'

Back at the farm the Sheriff counted the final tally – 208 birds, including twenty woodcock and several drakes. There they all were, their heads held between rows of nails. We could buy them for three pounds each but I had lost my appetite. While I'd loved the day out in the country with my new friends, enjoying the banter and the liquid refreshments, my toes were now on the critical list. I took a hot bath to thaw out but no matter how many times I dunked my head beneath the water I couldn't erase the memory of the Guns walking proudly towards the shoot wagon – four or five heads hooked between their fingers and a certain swagger in their walk.

It seemed to me that the appeal of this sport lay in demonstrating man's mastery over land and beast – the more pheasants killed the higher the status of the male. According to Desmond Morris, the anthropologist I'd done some work with back in The Advertising Years, 'status' was an ancient driver of men. I could hear his words, uttered in the comfort of his Oxford library, surrounded by his friend Picasso's work, and his own surreal paintings of biological misfits. 'You see, Lucy, the reason "Status" has survived so long as a funda-mental human driver is because every hierarchical group needs order and stability. Within such a group there is a struggle for social dominance and the leader must display certain trappings and behaviour.' This might, to a caveman, have been Raquel Welch in a fur bikini, now it might be a Porsche, a copy of *The Economist,* or perhaps a golden British Airways Executive Club badge dangling from a shoulder bag on the red-eye to New York. Wasn't shooting pheasants just another, though perhaps more authentic, expression of this ancient driver? It was only slightly tarnished by the fact that the pheasants were reared, which might be the equivalent of taking Viagra – it looked good but it wasn't a real test of skill.

For me the appeal lay in the day's fulfilment of another ancient driver, 'Tribalism'. 'The external world threw non-stop challenges in the face of the hunter,' explained Desmond, 'the result was a shift towards combining and sharing resources, for added strength and security.' Now that, the sound of sixteen flags swooshing through the air, the mutual aid of the hot-dog donation, the banter in the wagon, was, for me, worth preserving for all time.

Sadly I couldn't get over the killing bit and the search for my gang, a group of people whose emotional bread and butter was the same as mine, continued.

There was one other way to join a ready-made tribe. There were three churches near the farmhouse – actually there were two as one was a ruin – all that was left of All Saints was an ancient ivy-clad tower and a few overgrown tombs. The second was the Protestant St Mary's, which was built to serve the residents of the grand Jacobean hall that lay behind it, and there was the Catholic church, a hundred metres up the lane, built in the Italian style in the late nineteenth century by the then owner of the hall after a Road to Damascus conversion.

It was clear, from the first moment we saw Our Lady of Perpetual Succour, that David had found his tribe. We'd stood before it, one sunny Sunday back in July, taking in the grassy graveyard populated with ornate black wrought-iron crosses and the plain red-brick building with its twin turrets, arch windows and crowning glory – a stone statue of the Virgin Mary with child. David loved it and resolved to attend the next service – I thought I'd go too until I found out that it was held at eight on a Sunday morning. David had a commitment that had been handed down through the centuries – his ancestors come from Portuguese Goa, where Catholicism still thrives. I, on the other hand, went to a Quaker School that taught Human Studies in place of Religious Education and consequently I have the religious liberalism of many of my generation, pluralist and tolerant, believing in the idea of many paths, paths that all lead to one place, a place bigger than oneself, better than oneself, but not necessarily a place inhabited by a benevolent God looking down on our endeavours. I was definitely not used to there being One Way, the Catholic way – but eventually, following several weeks of rave reviews from David, I found myself getting out of bed, for the first time ever on a Sunday, at half past seven in the morning. It soon became a regular, one Sunday in three, or maybe four, thing.

It was a pretty whitewashed church with wrought-iron balustrades, a gold-trimmed dome, dark mahogany floorboards and simple wooden chairs. I liked the way that the congregation responded to David – he might have been the first Paki to worship in the church but they welcomed him with open arms, or at least with warm smiles and friendly nods in his direction. Now he was evidently one of them – a member of a broad church with no age or wage restrictions – there were lords and there were ladies, there were plumbers and there were roofers, there were little girls in bright pink jackets too excited to kneel, and there were trembling men of ninety who no longer could.

I'd sit quietly and reflect on the week that had been, enjoying the reassuringly timeless service. It felt good to take the time to stop and think about what we are doing on this earth; to hear about the pilgrimage to the shrine at Walsingham, to sponsor children so that they could attend the church's school in the Congo, to learn of the arrival of a parish computer 'ten years younger than the old one'. Listening to prayers for parishioners in hospital and for the starving in Africa reminded me that life might present bigger issues than what colour to paint our walls.

I'd met some charismatic holy men in India, some of them gave good *darshan* (audiences), but none of them compared to the Dom, whose wide-ranging and provocative homilies could encompass, in six minutes, what gets in the way of our ability to take the actions we know we should, our self-serving definitions of justice, and the reasons why prostitutes might enter the Kingdom of Heaven first. I am afraid that none of these homilies convinced me to become a Catholic, although all of them made me want to be a better person. They were David's favourite part of the service and he never lost an opportunity to suggest improvements to the Dom as we stood outside mingling with our fellow worshippers. The first few times it happened the Dom was receptive, happy to stand amongst the gravestones and discuss David's considerations. After that I noticed a cooling-off period in which the Dom would give him five minutes and then have urgent business to attend to, 'people to see, places to go, breakfast to eat, long morning ahead, busiest day of the week...' he'd cry as he rushed to his car clutching his Jesus Travels shoulder bag.

My favourite part of the service was giving each other 'the sign of peace' – 'peace be with you' we said as we smiled and shook hands with our pew neighbours, 'and also with you' came the reply; it was a chance to smile at strangers, to break down some of the barriers that stand between us – I found myself thinking that London would be a much better place if we walked around making the same gesture; such a small thing, but so uplifting.

When it came to taking communion I piously crossed my arms over my chest (signifying that I hadn't been confirmed a Catholic and would only require a blessing). I was a little surprised the first time I went to receive my blessing to find the Dom taking the opportunity to bash me over the head three times. I was so shocked all I could do was say 'Amen', get to my feet and walk away. In subsequent weeks I would tell him that my reluctance to convert dated from this habit of hitting me over the head but the truth was that despite the sense of community it offered, the sense of belonging, I just couldn't get past my own religious liberalism. While I loved the *idea* of believing in one God, the creator, he remained an *idea*. While David will tell you that he knows God and loves Him, I just know that I love the church, the people who go to that church, and the Dom.

Even though it was clear that Catholicism was never going to be my tribe the Dom soon became a friend; when he drove his battered old car through our gates it sent gravel flying and David to the drinks cabinet – David and I shared a private joke that he should be known as Dom Perignon. It wasn't just a shared love of good wine that drew us together, the Dom was excellent company and very funny – his wit was as dry as the desert, somewhat reminiscent of Stephen Fry, but cleverer and less pompous. It was a wit that had evidently found a receptive audience at Downside School where he'd been headmaster. I heard one anecdote in which he'd posted a note beside the plate of apples offered for pupils' consumption:

'Take only ONE. God is watching.'

At the other end of the table was a large pile of chocolate chip cookies, on which a pupil had written a note:

'Take all you want. God is watching the apples.'

He announced at a baptism that 'our insurance is up to date so we can give the children candles to hold', reminded us, when politicians told us to 'hug a hoodie', that 'monks have been hoodies for centuries', and never missed an opportunity to send up his own predilection for red wine – offering the congregation bottles in return for putting in good words with his boss, the Abbot.

One Saturday afternoon he popped round to bless our house. He was fresh from hearing the eco confessions of those who'd failed to recycle their bottles of Pinot Grigio in the Earthly Sins booth at the Waveney Greenpeace Festival and I was sorry that he'd changed out of his green chasuble made of recycled curtains, but perhaps he thought black would be more acceptable to us. I had imagined that this ceremony would take several hours and require David and I to say a few words – perhaps promising to love and cherish the farmhouse, for richer, for poorer, in sickness or in health, till death do us part. I imagined wrong. The Dom had a restorative cup of tea and a slice of Tesco Finest tarte au citron, which I may have passed off as my own (bless me, father, for I have sinned), we had a quick but immensely erudite (on his part) discussion around the great moral issue of the day (whether all parents love their children) until he jumped up suddenly, grabbed a jug, filled it with tap water and sprinkled it through the hall using a stalk of rosemary from the herb garden. There was a sentence involving the words 'bless this house' but I only caught the tail end because I was closing the back door behind us. Picking up his copy of the *Catholic Herald* he was gone in a sweep of cassock – probably to save the local outdoor swimming pool from closure, or to visit a troubled family in need of arbitration.

On the two Sundays in three that I wasn't at church I was generally practising yoga at home, maybe not on the dot of eight but certainly I was well underway by the time David had returned home with a cleansed soul. David told the Dom what I was doing and he pretended (I think) to be horrified. I was a bit worried that I might've caused offence so we invited him over – it was a good excuse to sink a glass or three, and perhaps driven by guilt at my non-attendance, and my desire to impress a Radio Four contributor, I determined to explain how yoga might actually benefit the practice of religion.

'Although it's come down to us via Buddhism, Jainism and Hinduism, yoga isn't specific to any one of those religions,' I began earnestly, 'as the Indian guru Osho said, "It was an accident that the Christians discovered physics and it was an accident that the Hindus discovered yoga".'

'That's right,' said David, refilling our glasses, 'yoga reaches beyond our beliefs as Catholics or Muslims or Hindus, and knowing that we are all the same on the inside, it focuses on internal transformation.'

'So it benefits anyone, of any religion,' I added enthusiastically, 'helping us get beyond the demands of our ego so that we can be a force for good in the world.'

The Dom smiled and nodded and politely refrained from pointing out that ten years of practising yoga hadn't yet turned me into such a force for good that I could be relied upon to turn up at church every Sunday.

'I read about a vicar who banned yoga classes in his church hall because he saw it as a New Age teaching and a threat to the Christian establishment,' I informed the Dom, 'he was worried that it would be a gateway into Eastern mysticism for his congregation.'

The Dom had no such concerns. 'My only objection is that it might, if taken to extremes, encourage a certain physical obsession which I don't see as healthy.

'However,' he concluded, contemplating his ample girth, 'I don't think I would be in any danger of that particular obsession.'

A couple of glasses later we said goodbye to our favourite priest, poured ourselves another drink and transferred ourselves to the sofa in front of the newly installed wood burner.

'Do you think the vicar's real problem with yoga was that the yoga classes were better attended than his services?' I suggested. 'I read recently that just under a million people attend church every Sunday, so I looked up how many go to yoga – it's staggering – more than 1.2 million go every week, and another 1.5 million say they go occasionally.'

'Wow,' said David, smiling at my continuing ability to spout numbers, a leftover from my advertising days when I always had to be ready to outline the latest statistics on a campaign's effectiveness to a client.

'Perhaps yoga has actually become a religion of sorts,' I suggested. 'Think about it, there's a discipline for every mind set: Ashtanga with its emphasis on regular practice seems closest to Catholicism, Iyengar's puritanical approach might be considered Protestant, the individualist yoga of Desikachar might be seen as Quaker liberalism.'

'Maybe,' he agreed, 'traditional religions, with their promises of reward after death, struggle in our age of instant gratification, but yoga, with its fast delivery of buff bodies and mental calm in stressful times, has plenty of relevance to today. But it's not just yoga – the pursuit of youth is the real twenty-first-century religion – everyone wants to look younger and yoga is just one way to get there.'

I thought yoga's appeal also had to do with the sense of community it offers. David disagreed: 'Yoga is appealing because it gives you a Brad Pitt fit body and helps you look younger – for most people it's just a physical thing, nothing to do with community. They just come, do their practice and go.'

'But what about The Cappuccino Gurus?' I argued. 'I met them through yoga and now they're my closest friends.'

'You met them on a yoga holiday, that's different. You spent time with each other, you got to know each other, you drank too much Rioja...'

'Well okay, the holiday was the catalyst, but it could've gone the way of a holiday romance, exciting at the time and fizzling out shortly afterwards, but we've met regularly ever since, and...'

'... and what?'

'Of course,' I said, slapping my forehead. 'Why didn't I think of it before? I can't go on cruising Tesco at nine at night, simply to see people other than the ones on my TV screen – I'll join a local yoga class. I'm sure I'll find some like-minded souls there – The Cappuccino Gurus of the East – and if that doesn't happen at least I'll get Brad Pitt fit.'

'Cool, Babe,' said David, pouring me another glass of Rioja.

7

'The dog was having its balls chopped off'

Even if I didn't meet The Cappuccino Gurus of the East I would, I reasoned, feel less alone in a room full of like-minded folk. This strategy had worked when I was on business in Delhi, New York or Milan – exhausted and missing David, the familiarity of the postures had helped me to feel at home in the city – to paraphrase Paul Young, 'wherever I throw my mat that's my home'. Even if I didn't understand the local language I could be confident I would understand the teacher because he or she would name the *asana* or postures in Sanskrit, a language that had been handed down through many generations, to become the universal vocabulary of yoga.

Yoga classes also gave me a rare proximity to the locals; I enjoyed the Central Park studio where I could be sure of rubbing shoulders with the Park Avenue Princesses – let's face it, putting my mat down next to Ms Bergdorf was the closest I was going to get to being her neighbour. I squeezed in super-strong classes with the tattooed 'liberated while living' crowd at Jivamukti's downtown studio, coming home with 'everything one needs for a yogic lifestyle' from their eco-friendly fair trade organic boutique. I spent a Sunday morning at a yoga class in a hip neighbourhood of LA, delighting in the Eric Clapton soundtrack and my mat neighbour who had a film script by her side. She was blonde and skinny. Was it Gwyneth? Nicole? Lindsay? I was practically a member of Hollywood.

Finding a class in New York or Los Angeles was easy – there were yoga centres everywhere and the classes were all drop in, easy come, easy go. The same could not be said of Norfolk. I tried the British Wheel of Yoga's website and *Eco Echo*, the free magazine listing everything alternative in the county, but I spoke to a dozen teachers before I found one who didn't have a long waiting list. The problem seemed to be the size of the venues – theatre rehearsal rooms, arts centre studios, attics – most of them could only fit ten or twelve people at a time, and students secured their place by signing up for nine or ten-week terms, paying in advance. So, when Sandra announced that she did have a place in her class, I felt as if I had just scored tickets to see Led Zeppelin at the O2.

'I should just warn you,' said Sandra, 'in this area yoga is more for older people. It means that the practice is generally slower, less physically demanding. I suggest that you do some Ashtanga classes in Norwich for your physical needs and use my classes for pranayama and meditation.'

'That's okay, ' I said confidently, 'I am pretty old myself and I am trying to relax to get pregnant, so a softer, more opening practice is more appropriate for me right now.'

The hall wasn't quite what I'd been used to – in place of Triyoga's stained-glass windows and a Zen white ceiling there were nine electric heaters suspended from the ceiling, and a disco ball. The heaters were just as well, it was getting on for the end of October and it was freezing. I put down my mat, noticing that the yoga student accessories were somewhat different to those of the Primrose Hill set – one of my neighbours had an industrial-strength bright yellow torch and the other, Edith, had a vast spade – she'd brought it to lend to one of the other ladies who had to tackle some big weeds in the garden.

We arranged ourselves around the room; the sight of a row of older ladies with tartan blankets wrapped over outstretched legs, silk scarves carefully arranged to keep heads and necks warm, made me smile – reminding me of a day out in a vintage open-topped car. The ten women clearly knew each other well, chatting so intensely it was hard for Sandra, a skinny woman clad entirely in black apart from her head which was wrapped in a hippy's rainbow cloth bandana, to get the class started. I didn't mind – I enjoyed listening to their banter:

'You're complaining again, Edith!'

'Ah,' said Edith, adjusting her scarf, 'you wouldn't recognise me if I wasn't complaining.

'Did anyone go to St Michael's weddings and flowers exhibition last week?' she asked, 'I was away so I missed it – such a shame.'

It was universally agreed to have been another triumph for the local flower guilds.

There was a long discussion about who should've won the Women's Institute tiddlywinks contest, and then they moved on to Edith's much-anticipated performance in a forthcoming Gilbert and Sullivan production, which was universally predicted to be a triumph.

Eventually we got down to business, starting gently, with Child's Pose, kneeling with our head on the floor, our arms by our sides.

'I find this pose so uncomfortable – it's my spare tyre – it seems to have got bigger,' said Edith, sitting up and lifting her jumper for us to have a look.

We all duly looked and some of us made efforts to dispute the size of the tyre but another lady stepped in before we got ourselves into too much trouble.

'Does that mean you'll definitely be coming with us to the belly dancing workshop next week, Edith?' she quipped.

Everyone was sixty plus, and Sandra's warning that this would be a slow and gentle class was well founded. The lady on the mat next to me sucked and swallowed her way through the next hour and a half, commanding a great deal of Sandra's attention as she hauled her painfully arthritic body into each pose. Sandra ministered to her with the tenderness of Florence Nightingale but clearly the elderly woman was really hurting.

We'd been given a so-called Angel Card by Edith at the beginning of the practice. It was, she explained, 'an inspiring message for the class, something to keep in your mind'. My card was entitled 'Understanding' and I tried to remind myself that stiffness teaches us to be where we are, to fully experience the journey into each pose. But my flexibility and fitness were hard won, I'd spent ten years practising yoga three or four times a week, and I didn't want to lose everything that I'd worked for. What would happen to me if I only did this class? Would I end up reverting to my pre-yoga state – unable to reach the floor? I didn't want to throw all that work away. My stepmother Nikki had told me that my figure had changed almost completely in the time I'd been practising yoga and I have to admit to a certain vanity in wanting to retain it – especially if I were to get pregnant and spend the next nine months expanding in all sorts of directions. I knew it was good for me to learn to relax, but I really struggled to stay in the room – an hour later and we'd only done four or five poses. We then spent half an hour on breathing exercises, urged to listen only to what was in the room and immediately outside. I tried to focus on the wind whipping around the hall walls and roof but to be completely honest all I could think about was running screaming for the hills. Perhaps 'Be Here Now' would have been a more appropriate Angel Card for me. Though I knew this was exactly the kind of class I needed to do I also knew I wouldn't be coming back. I just couldn't hack the feeling that I might be in heaven's waiting room.

A 'Yoga meets Qigong' class was no more to my taste. The teacher told me on the phone that the class would involve traditional *asana* with flowing movements plus the directed breathing of Qigong, a practice normally found in Taoist and Buddhist monasteries as an adjunct to martial arts training – usually under a strict teacher–disciple relationship. I imagined her as a *Crouching Tiger, Hidden Dragon* warrior, brandishing a sword, pursuing thieves across rooftops and forests dressed in a golden cape, jet black hair scraped back into a bun held together with chopsticks.

She turned out to be a well-spoken white-haired sixty-something in old green cords and a comfortable white Aran jumper. We met at six in the complementary health centre reception, beneath the rafters of the converted barn, rafters steeped in years of aromatherapy and incense. She welcomed everyone as they arrived and we sat comfortably on the large sofas drinking green tea and making a fuss of the centre's huge furry dog. Fido decided to make a beeline for my lap, its size forming a screen that effectively cut me out of all conversation. Perhaps it was just as well – I didn't think I would've been able to contribute much; my fellow class-mates were mostly yummy mummies – the car park had been crowded with 4x4s and here they were, resplendent in Boden's vibrant polka-dot-lined lightweight wool coats and matching wellies, exchanging points of view on the relative merits of local schools and children's party entertainers. I wondered what Gabriele would've made of the scene before me – I suspected that they were rather less competitive than their counterparts in north-west London.

The class took place in a pretty room decorated in pale blue with framed photographs of planet earth on the walls. We settled down on two rows of mats facing each other, the teacher sat in the middle adjusting her large jumper and cords, checking we were all warm enough. We were, and so we began. The promisingly titled Immortality Sequence turned out to be a slow standing forward bend followed by a slow stretch upwards. The idea, she explained, was to 'die in the moment and be reborn'. We scooped imaginary water with our hands – right then left. We pretended we were holding a beach ball, passing it backwards and forwards. We performed one slow sun salutation. I was all for softness, and definitely all for immortality, but I was moving so slowly I began to worry that I might die in the moment and not have the energy to be reborn. Once more I wanted to run screaming for the hills – but instead I just about made it to the end of the class, then I ran screaming for the car and never went back.

*

I'd tried every yoga teacher I could find within easy travelling distance of the farmhouse and I was running out of options. What to do? I fled to Norwich (population 367,035) for the only known antidote – some fast-moving Ashtanga yoga. I'd always found it too fast paced but I suddenly found myself craving a racing heart and a sweat – at least I'd know I was alive.

This is how I found myself knocking at the door of The Lotus Room, opposite the Mecca bingo hall and next to John Lewis, forming a spiritual golden triangle. The door flew open and I found myself in the arms of a tiny mischievous imp, a human fireball of energy clad in bright pink leggings and an orange vest top.

Kiki hugged me until I could no longer breathe.

When we finally let go of each other I was able to take in the details – the tanned and sculpted yoga body, the sun-streaked mane of hair that tumbled around her shoulders, the pale green eyes, the radiant smile. She wore not a trace of make-up and I thought her utterly beautiful.

We'd only spoken once before – when I'd rung to find out whether she had room in her class for me; having ascertained that I was the Lucy Edge whose book she'd read she confessed that she had a funny story to tell me. 'So, my horrible ex-boyfriend went to Mysore to study with Pattabhi Jois,' explained Kiki. 'I didn't hear from him for a while and then I found out that he'd gone off with a girl called Lucy who was writing a book about yoga in Mysore and, when I saw your book, I was convinced it was you. I looked up your website and there was a picture of you taking a dip in the Ganges, looking blissed-out and wholesome; I couldn't understand what you saw in him – he's horrible!'

'Well, *you* went out with him…' I countered, teasing her.

'Anyway, finally I spoke to someone who knew you and,' said Kiki with evident relief, 'she assured me that it wasn't you.'

I was relieved too – it already felt as if we would be friends and I didn't want anything to get in the way. Still, I had my own confession to make. 'Kiki, I have to be honest,' I said, looking at the floor, 'the truth is that I probably would've run off with him if he'd shown any interest but I don't think I met him and anyway, I lived a life of unwanted celibacy the whole time I was there. I couldn't score for love or money.'

'Well,' continued Kiki gleefully, 'the other Lucy dumped him a year later so he got what he deserved.'

United by the certain knowledge that karma was a wonderful thing we went through double doors to the yoga studio, a peaceful sunny room enriched with the deep rooted smell of incense. To the side of a golden dais garlanded with big pink plastic flowers sat a framed photograph of Ashtanga guru Pattabhi Jois, and in front of the dais were twelve pink and orange yoga mats on which were already perched nine young women and two men, all ready to get down to business. I took my place on the remaining mat and felt immediately at home.

Kiki prepared her iPod which rested on a huge portable loudspeaker. How the heck did she lug that around? The girl didn't need a boyfriend, she needed a roadie.

'I'm hit by a sudden desire to play the theme from the *A Team*,' said Kiki mischievously. 'Do I hear any other requests?'

'"Don't Stop Movin'" by S Club 7?' I suggested.

'Hmm,' said Kiki thoughtfully – not sure I have that one. Maybe some Spice Girls? I was having a night of *Guilty Pleasures* with my daughters last night – we danced till dawn to David Essex and Dolly Parton.'

In the end we settled for some *Mystic India* chants – one of my favourites.

It was a challenging class – exactly what I needed – fast moving with lots of variations – none of which I could do but at least I could watch other people doing them, and for once that made me feel good – inspired even. Then I had a horrible thought – did these young yogis feel the same way about me as I did about the old-timers in Sandra's classes? Think about it – the age difference was about the same – these women were all in their twenties. I was in my forties. The 'old-timers' in Sandra's class were in their sixties. Were these young women irritated by my inability to do *Parsva Bakasana*, or Sideways Crane, in which both thighs rested on the back of an upper arm, while the head lifted effortlessly off the floor? Did they worry that my stiffness might be catching? Was I making wheezing noises? Did I snore in *Savasana*? Perhaps I should take a leaf out of Edith's book and hand round some 'Understanding' Angel Cards.

After the class Kiki asked me if I would like to go to a birthday party with her on Saturday night. Sadly I couldn't make it but it got us talking about age.

'I'm forty-three,' she announced, smiling.

I was horrified. She couldn't be the same age as me. She had few wrinkles and the buff body of a twenty-five-year-old. She could rest both her thighs on the back of an elbow. She would easily have won the unofficial body-fat contests in Mysore in which the yoga students pumped and preened poolside as they displayed bodies that hadn't had to deal with a jam doughnut since they went macrobiotic ten years previously. Except that something told me Kiki was the kind of girl who would eat a jam doughnut with the same degree of relish as me.

'And I've got three children,' she added.

'And how old are they?' I asked nervously.

'My twin girls are eighteen, they're taking a gap year to travel this year, they leave for India next week, and then next year they'll go to university as medical students,' she said proudly. 'My son is ten,' she added, clearly enchanted by the mere mention of him.

I wondered what I'd been doing with my life.

As we were leaving I asked Kiki if she knew of any teachers more local to me and she suggested that I try Kate – another Lotus Room teacher who held a vinyasa flow class in Beccles on a Wednesday night. 'You'll love her, Lucy, she looks just like Kate Hudson and she's a Bad Lady, just like me.'

'What's a Bad Lady, Kiki?' I asked. I thought I might know but I just wanted to check.

'A Bad Lady has it going on, Lucy,' she said, rotating her arms and hips in the manner of a *Jerry Springer* participant. 'A Bad Lady works hard, she's good at what she does, she knows who she is, but she doesn't take life too seriously – all her hard work is balanced with lots of yoga, lots of friends, lots of workshops on men, lots of dancing, and lots and lots of Pinot Grigio.'

She could've been describing me. I smiled broadly, very relieved to hear about the Pinot Grigio consumption. I told her that I'd been worried that she might've been a bit of an

Ashtanga nut. David joked that Ashtangis were not just the Catholics of the yoga world, they were the Jesuits – the hard-core element of the yoga fraternity; those yogic overachievers who eat only macrobiotic Edamame beans, go to bed at nine so they can practise at dawn, and eschew alcohol in favour of organic carrot juice.

'God no,' said Kiki, 'nothing could be further from the truth. I am such a Bad Lady I even write an occasional blog called Two Bad Ladies with an American girl I met in Mysore,' she continued. 'It's about a medicated and moti-vated Ashtanga teacher with "Dolce e Gabbana" tattooed in Sanskrit across her shoulder blades.'

'Sounds brilliant,' I declared, making a note of the blog address. 'I'm also an official Bad Lady – I did a workshop with Pattabhi Jois in London and that's what he called me when he saw my collapsing *Chaturanga Dandasana*. Then I nearly toppled him when he was holding my foot out to the right and I lost my balance. I was so embarrassed I decided to study with someone else when I went to Mysore.'

'Oh, you shouldn't have worried about it,' said Kiki consolingly. 'We're all "Bad Ladies" in his mind. Anyway, enjoy meeting Kate and why don't the three of us go out for a drink next week? It'll be a "Yogutante" coming-out party for the latest addition to the ranks of Norfolk's Bad Ladies,' she said, authoritatively.

I rang Kate the next morning and just before eight that very Wednesday evening I found myself parking in Beccles Market Square to the peal of St Michael's church bells. I walked through the square and turned off into the Quaker Meeting House's courtyard, a peaceful refuge which was somehow hermetically sealed from the sound of traffic only feet away. The pretty building, comprising two eighteenth-century Dutch gabled cottages, formed an L shape around the court-yard. In the corner of the L was a blackboard on which were chalked three arrows; I got a bit overexcited when I thought the one pointing left read 'Swingers' – but as I got closer it became 'Singers'. The singers had already started work – the strains of Gilbert and Sullivan's *Pirates of Penzance* spilling out of the windows; 'I am the very model of a modern Major General,' sang the Major General. I wondered if I should alert my mum, she'd performed in *The Mikado* to great critical acclaim. The arrow pointing right read 'Knit and Knatter' – this was clearly a well-attended meeting judging by the volume of laughter coming from the room. A grey-haired lady stood outside with her friend, explaining that there had been a raffle to raise money for the Mayor's Appeal and a cheque for £85 was being presented to the mayoress that evening. Just at that moment the mayoress herself arrived and the three ladies bustled past me, clutching their handbags to their stom-achs. I wished I could clone myself and attend, I'd never been very good at knitting and I thought I might learn a thing or two, but I had a date with destiny; I followed the arrow for 'Yoga', it pointed in an upwards direction.

The door was shut so I sat on the stairs and waited for ten minutes. Slowly the stairs filled up with my fellow students – a sixteen-year-old with a mass of tumbling black hair and pouting lips, her friend who remained silent but who smiled in the manner of a cherub, a brown-as-a-berry thirty-something, a twenty-five-year-old woman with tattoos and a sprightly sixty-ish lady in a powder blue tracksuit. By the end of our wait I'd established that the two sixteen-year-olds were at the local school and that this was their first class with Kate, that the tattooed woman was a baker who'd apparently just won an award for her ginger cake, that the brown-as-a-berry thirty-something had a couple of children, had travelled round India on an Enfield motorbike and now lived in Great Yarmouth, and that the lady in the tracksuit worked for a charity shop in Beccles and had been coming to Kate's classes for years.

Eventually the door to the yoga room burst open and six women tumbled out giggling.

'We thought you were all deep in *Savasana*,' I said. It was a long time to be in Corpse Pose but maybe it had been a tough class.

'Nope, just gossiping,' they admitted, bursting into another fit of giggles and bundling down the stairs.

Something told me this was going to work out.

We gathered up our mats and bags and went in. It may have had stained-glass windows of red and yellow comparable to Triyoga's blue, turquoise and orange panes of glass but in every other way the small room was substantially different; it had the appearance of an old aunt's sitting room – a carriage clock on the mantelpiece, standard lamps with chintz shades, and a plant growing out of a teapot.

Kate sat calmly at the end of the room, a serene willowy slip of a woman in dove-grey yoga pants and a gypsy style white flowing top over which embroidered butterflies flew. If Kiki was a hot summer's sun this girl was a full moon on a winter's night. Kiki was right, she looked just like Hollywood actress Kate Hudson; loose waves of silvery blonde hair shimmered in the evening light, her pale skin glowed, her grey eyes shone as big as saucers.

She smiled a mega-watt smile that lit up the room more effectively than all the candles with which she was surrounded.

'Welcome,' she said, bowing her head gently, effortlessly adjusting her lithe and limber frame into lotus position.

The youngest girls took the front row and I put my mat down between the brown-as-a-berry girl and the sprightly sixty-something.

It was a blissful class – carefully sequenced and conducted at a measured pace, it was clear that Kate took her teaching very seriously. I found it hard to remember what we'd done afterwards because it had a dream-like quality, an hour and a half covered in a soft haze, washed down by a chilled Café Del Mar soundtrack delivered on an antique CD ghetto blaster, only occasionally interrupted by bursts of enthusiasm from the *Pirates of Penzance* rehearsals down below. There'd been some sun salutations, some 'dancing warriors', some sliding of hands down thighs and reaching of hands to the sky – or at least towards the two giant paper lantern lampshades above. There'd been some circular movements which utilised every corner of the mat, some forward bends and some back bends, some shoulder stands. But the finer details were a complete loss to me. How did we get from A to B? No idea. It was as if I'd entered a yogic Bermuda Triangle – I wasn't quite sure what had gone on there, but there was something quite magical about it.

We bowed our heads to thank her and eventually I managed to make my way to my feet and get out my chequebook. Kate smiled warmly and refused to take any payment – 'the first class is free of charge,' she said, waving away my money. In all the classes I'd ever done it was the first time I'd come across a try-before-you-buy policy – I liked it.

'Kiki told me she was organising a Yogutante party for you,' said Kate, packing away her many yoga blocks and mats.

'Yes, she's hoping we can get together on Tuesday night,' I replied, 'do her class and then go for a bite to eat. I can't remember the name of the restaurant, I'm afraid.'

'Baba Ghanoush?'

'That's the one.'

'Yes, that's our usual spot for après yoga,' said Kate, laughing.

'You do après yoga?' I asked, my eyes widening with incredulity.

'Of course,' said Kate, 'what's the point of yoga without the après?'

I couldn't believe my luck. My heart leapt. I had definitely found my tribe.

I emerged into the courtyard at the same time as the Knit and Knatter gang, led by a happy-looking mayoress. For a moment I was swept up in their swarming chatter; I nodded and smiled and clutched my yoga mat to my chest, just as they carried their handbags. Looking up at the black night and the stars above I thanked each one, unable to believe that I'd finally met my gang, and discovered two fantastic yoga teachers, all in the space of twenty-four hours.

The Yogutante party happened the following Tuesday after Kiki's class. Kate did the class too, there we were – two Bad Ladies mat to mat – except that I seemed to be the only one who was really bad. I was an immediate admirer of Kate's graceful drop backs, those silvery blonde waves of hers tickling her ankles, and her effortless handstand, which she performed unsupported in the middle of the room as I struggled to launch myself against the wall. She balanced in Sideways Crane, apparently Kiki's favourite pose, both thighs tucked neatly onto the back of her upper arm, her head lifted effortlessly off the floor. I hoped that her flexibility and strength might be catching, it certainly inspired me to try, even if I did crash-land on my nose.

After the class we got changed behind wooden screens erected for the purpose – in went Kate's yoga chick comprising a stripy ballet jumper and black trousers, out came Ibiza Girl. Wearing an off-the-shoulder floral top belted low on the hips, flared pale blue jeans covered in patches and espadrilles, a silk rose pinned to the side of her head, she would've been quite at home on Salinas beach, swaying her pale slender limbs to lazy Balearic beats in the hazy afternoon sun. Kiki went behind the screen wearing her signature pink and orange and emerged as a forties film star – in a vintage olive-green tea dress that perfectly matched her eyes, accessorised with a matching clutch bag and T-bar shoes with a scalloped back and two-inch heels. I looked down at my outfit and sighed, I'd always felt comfortable in what *Vogue* magazine might've termed 'haute gap year' – jeans, boots, big belt and hippy beads – but compared to them I was a Yoga Yokel. I noticed with dismay that my boots weren't even clean – they were battered and spattered with mud – next to these girls I might as well have had straw in my hair and a rucksack made of tie-dyed hemp.

We walked slowly to the restaurant from The Lotus Room, it was half past seven and there were only a few people around to brave the cold. I wondered how Kate was doing in her espadrilles and off-the-shoulder top but she seemed to be warmed by that mega-watt smile of hers. The three Bad Ladies linked arms, me in the middle, as they led me past the stripy awnings of the closed-up stalls in the market square, down an alley way, and up a staircase, where we emerged into a warm candlelit room that felt like an attic. We sat at a table by a window that offered us a simultaneous view of St John's Maddermarket church and Spearmint Rhino strip club and immediately ordered a bottle of Pinot Grigio.

The girls were keen to know about my transition from London to the countryside and to my surprise (it normally takes me quite a while to share the personal stuff) I found myself giving them the full monty – I explained how I'd got weary of London and come to Norfolk with a somewhat romantic notion of country life; how I'd envisaged children's picnics in fields of poppies, plentiful recycling of vintage cashmere, much making of home-made jam. I outlined what I'd been doing in the name of fertility – I'd given up coffee (completely), I'd given up drinking (nearly), and I'd been learning to relax (sometimes).

'What else can I do?'

'Have you thought about yoga for fertility?' suggested Kate, ordering a selection of Baba Ghanoush's specials for the three of us. 'I know someone who specialises in it, why don't you try her?'

She turned out to be in London, and I really wanted a local teacher.

'What about getting the information from a book? There's one called *Luna Yoga*,' suggested Kate again, 'I came across it on my British Wheel of Yoga training and it's all about fertility. I'll bring it to class tomorrow.'

I thanked her and we moved on to other discoveries – that Kiki had a new love interest.

'I met him a couple of weeks ago on a yoga and surf weekend in Devon,' explained Kiki. 'He was the surf instructor and I was teaching yoga. He's absolutely gorgeous – all rippling torso and long bronzed limbs and…'

'How old is he, Kiki?' asked Kate, passing around the endless supply of Mediterranean mezze that had just arrived at our table.

'Umm, I think he's in his early thirties.'

'Go, girl,' said Kate, laughing.

'Anyway, we stayed up late one night talking about wedging A-frames and the quest for the perfect wave and we ended up having a snog,' said Kiki, smiling like the cat that'd got the cream. 'I don't know how much he's got between his ears but with a body like his who cares? I think he's going to come up for a weekend soon – he wants to try surfing off the east-Norfolk coast.'

I was as intrigued by Kiki's clothes as I was by her love life and asked her where they came from; it turned out that she was a regular in the vintage quarter of Norwich, combing the rails for dresses that cast her as a film-noir heroine. She may have looked like a twenty-five-year-old but her glamorous shoes were the kind it takes a woman with experience to appreciate. She'd picked them up in Buenos Aires where she'd spent a month learning the Argentine Tango.

'Every time I saw a pair of shoes I loved on the dance floor I'd ask the girl wearing them where they were from and they'd turn out to be from the same designer. It was really hard to track him down – he doesn't advertise, has no website or catalogue but eventually I found a girl who was willing to introduce me. I came back with ten pairs.'

It turned out that Kiki had been a dancer before she became a yoga goddess – she'd gone to her first yoga class in her late twenties because she needed to stretch out her muscles after a particularly gruelling performance – and a decade later had become a full-time yoga teacher. She'd gone to Buenos Aires to get some inspiration for her PhD on the relationship between yoga, breath and dance, and had been very impressed with the level of talent on display in the dance halls. It seemed to me she could write another PhD on the courtship rituals she witnessed there – they sounded very complicated.

'A woman sits at a table in the hall but she can't dance until she catches the eye of the man,' she explained. 'She signifies her interest by holding his gaze, giving him The Look, and he will then come over and ask her to dance.'

'What if he isn't someone you want to dance with?' I asked, intrigued.

'Then it's quite simple; you mustn't catch his eye.'

'But what if you catch it accidentally?' asked Kate, laughing.

'You mustn't,' said Kiki, simply.

'But isn't that quite difficult?' I asked. 'What if you are just looking around and your eyes happen to land on this old man with no teeth?'

'Yes, but you learn how to not look, and how to Look, if you know what I mean.'

'So what does The Look look like?' I asked.

Kiki gave us a demonstration which started with a small bob of the head in a downwards direction, and was followed by a slow lift and then a direct gaze, the nature of which made me blush. This girl was obviously a very Bad Lady.

Kate had met her husband Will in slightly less romantic circumstances, in a Polish school where they'd both been working as teachers, teaching English as a foreign language.

'He proposed to me across the operating table,' she confided.

'Were you really ill?' I asked, imagining a romantic deathbed scenario carved out of a Hollywood movie.

'Oh no,' she replied, laughing heartily, 'the dog was having its balls chopped off.'

They'd married at the sixteenth-century grey flint country house I often admired on my riverfront walks in Beccles and they'd honeymooned an hour away, at an award-winning boutique hotel with an organic vegetable garden, low-energy light bulbs and lavatory cisterns fitted with hippos made from recycled plastic bottles to reduce water consumption. Now they lived in Harleston, a few miles south of Beccles, in a semi-detached house. 'We've only got a small garden but we've got an allotment and Will grows most of what we eat.'

'So you're Tom and Barbara from *The Good Life*,' I said laughing, 'it sounds idyllic.'

'It's not quite the picture of perfection you might imagine,' she confessed. 'Money can be tight, Will's a conservation officer so that doesn't pay a lot, and I don't earn much either. I teach eight yoga classes a week and I do monthly workshops at The Lotus Room but I've had to take a part-time admin job – it's not the job I was born to do but it pays the rent so I can enjoy teaching yoga without worrying too much about the money. I'm not in it to get rich, and I've got no ambition to move to London and teach there, but I'd hate to be in a position where I had to worry about the number of people in my classes.'

'It's not as easy to make money in Norfolk as it is in London,' explained Kiki. 'When I was living there I had a great job as a journalist which paid really well but here it's more about survival – people have to do the work that pays the bills, even if it's not what they would've chosen, and find ways to do what they love in their spare time.'

'Although there's a distinct absence of corporate ladders in the countryside, what we lose in vertical progress we make up for horizontally,' added Kate.

'But even making horizontal progress can be frustrating,' I said, 'especially now that the harvesting is done and the produce is being taken to the farms; it makes the slow roads even slower. When the bus got stuck behind a Waveney Mushrooms truck doing twenty miles an hour all the way to Norwich this afternoon I had to work really hard to remind myself that there's no point in having a heart attack on the way to a yoga class.'

'What I mean by horizontal progress is that local loyalty runs high and communities are tight knit,' explained Kate.

'Tell me about it,' I said, sighing, 'I've been at it for five months now and I'm still finding it hard to get involved. There's one couple who have been incredibly generous and kind, introducing us to all their friends, and we're friendly with the local priest but we've rather stalled since then.'

'Well, you have us now, Lucy,' said Kiki, raising her glass to mine. 'To our new Bad Lady,' she said. 'We love you already.'

We clinked glasses and I knew that I had at last found my emotional bread and butter.

*

On the bus home, my philosophical tendencies stirred by a couple of glasses of wine, I realised that I could detect a Pinot Grigio supping, smoking, or in some other way fundamentally flawed Bad Lady at a hundred paces – I'd been at the *Sivananda* ashram in Kerala for all of ten minutes when I came across Astrid and Cartier smuggling *Krishna*-endorsed *beedis* (tobacco wrapped in leaves) and a hip flask out of the ashram. They were my new best friends less than twenty-four hours later and I was still in touch with them now, five years later. Poppy shared my weaknesses for handbags, heels, Pinot Grigio and emotionally unavailable men, Gabriele smoked and liked a glass of wine, though her impeccable French taste ran a little higher than mine. Only thoroughly organic Andrea had no known vices, though perhaps her online dating adventures would lead her into some previously unknown territory. I smiled as I imagined the day of her corruption and wondered if I could organise a celebratory picture; all my Bad Ladies draped around the Ashtanga guru Pattabhi Jois. He would be cast as the artist formerly known as P. Diddy, bare-chested in a crisp white linen dhoti, several thick gold chains around his neck. My bad-ass girls would be covered in bling, they'd be drinking Cristal champagne and showing off their yoga-honed figures in bottom-hugging shorts, tiny Tees and Louboutins as they got jiggy to Frances's new album of Sanskrit chants – something of a departure from her favoured torch songs.

I wondered what it was about yoga that made me want to be bad. It seemed to be to do with seeing yoga as an essentially 'good thing' that had to be balanced out with some bad stuff – some small act of rebellion to help even out life's chances. Whatever the reason I was definitely not of the Jesuit school of yoga – I didn't want to set myself strict rules, to struggle with a four in the morning call to my mat, to become a yoga warrior. I knew that I wouldn't be able to win because I would be fighting myself – I had a feeling that trying too hard to be good would be exhausting, and the exhausted me would lose out to the bad part which would go into hiding, and like a terrorist cell, she would gather energy and eventually take me over completely. No, it was better to embrace the Bad Lady, to clasp her to my bosom and hold her tight, knowing that held close she couldn't do too much bad shit.

8

'Does my Uddiyana Bandha look big in this?'

I revisited the Beccles Quaker Meeting House the very next night; I was glad of a more gentle class following the rigours of Kiki's Ashtanga the night before, which had left me feeling more than a little stiff. The precise content of Kate's Wednesday class remained a mystery to me that night and for ever after – all I can say is that it was a seamless flow of postures that used up all four corners of the mat and disoriented me to the point that I forgot myself, except for the odd burst of laughter coming from the Knit and Knatter gang or a blast of Gilbert and Sullivan, until I was delivered promptly back to my mat bang on 9.30.

Kate and I went for a drink after the class, to The Swan House, a bar and restaurant at the centre of the market square run by Roland, a sixty-something Austrian-Russian-English Hornsey Arts School graduate come graphic designer come restaurateur, and his vivacious southern Italian partner Carmela. They'd remodelled the building, parts of which pre-dated 1540, for the twenty-first century with a vibe inspired by their favourite place – The Chelsea Arts Club. It was by far the most chilled-out spot in Beccles –

shabby chic furniture on the floor, a succession of local art on the walls and an eclectic mix of lesser-known gospel, blues, soul, folk and jazz on the iPod. Roland's taste in music was so good I suggested, more than once, that he sell it as a compilation, working title *The Swan Sessions*.

We peeled off layers of coats and scarves and settled down on one of the sofas in front of the roaring fire, ordered a glass of wine each, and a treacle tart to share. My step-father Oliver, not one for overdoing praise, was a big fan of The Swan's treacle tart – the first time he'd encountered it he'd eaten it in silence, pushed his empty plate away and announced thoughtfully that 'If there were inspectors of treacle tart then this one would win the top prize.' I could see him in that role – motoring around the country in a beaten-up Fiesta, the exhaust shaking and the fan belt whining and him not noticing – a man with a purpose; winding his way down narrow lanes to out-of-the-way pubs with nursery food menus. Arriving at his destination he'd reach for his clipboard and straighten his tie, sniffing portentously, his Roman nose held high; 'Good day to you, sir, I am here to check on the quality of your treacle tarts. Would you be so kind as to show me to a table?' There would be lots of columns on his clipboard – and room for erudite comments which would make good use of his Oxford degree and more recent Anglo-Saxon studies.

I digress.

I thanked Kate for the class and told her how much I'd enjoyed The Bad Ladies' night out, and that got us on to musing on the reasons why friendships formed through yoga feel so easy.

I had a theory. 'I think it's partly to do with the fact that in the practice of yoga we don't want anything from each other.' I expanded on my theme. 'The yoga mat is like an economic exclusion zone – in ten years of practising no one has ever asked me for anything more than to go for a glass of wine after class, and if economics does exist it works in our favour – you know I think there might be something of an emerging yoga mafia, in which we look after our own.'

Kate agreed and had some other theories.

'You feel a common thread immediately,' she said. 'You know everyone is there because they want to be a better person. Plus,' Kate joked, 'we're always opening our heart and throat *chakras* in class – no wonder we're so inclined to bond afterwards.'

Was the bonding process also held together by the tears that come with opening up the mind and body? 'I spent a yoga holiday at Ulpotha, an organic farm and yoga village in Sri Lanka, crying for three days solid,' I confessed, sipping my Pinot Grigio. 'And it wasn't because there wasn't a mini bar in my room. Actually, despite the notable absence of alcohol, it was one of the best holidays of my life, not just because we all learned a Britney Spears dance routine from a Hollywood star, but because it was on that holiday that I plucked up the courage to leave my job in advertising, the one where I'd been doing maternity cover for two women as well as my own job.'

'That's funny, I had a similar experience just recently,' said Kate. 'Do you know of Shiva Rea?'

I certainly did, I'd done a workshop with her at Triyoga and the woman had whisked me up into a handstand with a flick of her fingers. She was awesome, a Californian yoga goddess with a lion's mane of golden hair.

'I did her retreat on the island of Skyros last summer – everyone was in tears at least once over the course of the week, including me,' admitted Kate. 'And here's the weird thing, I loved every minute of it. It's such a relief to let go of all the shit, of all the anger, frustration and sadness that get in the way of our bliss on this planet. It's impossible to hold onto all that tension when the energy flows – it's like turning on a tap, all the crap in the sink gets washed away.'

'And by the time we've finished sobbing in the corner, by the time yoga has finished flushing out our ego, there's nowhere to hide anymore,' I said, 'so we might as well be truthful about our experiences and have a good laugh about it. It makes for some strong friendships – it's like there's no bullshit anymore.'

I told her how I was still in touch with Astrid and Cartier, my Yoga India tribe. 'We bonded over the production of a Nativity play directed by a man who spent his spare time on the phone to the porn stars of London, persuading them to lend their considerable expertise to a docudrama about spit-roasting footballers. We left the ashram together to spend a week travelling around Kerala, played a spliff-fuelled "Shoot, Shag or Marry?" on a houseboat and wished for bigger boobs in the human furnace that is the Hugging Mother, a living saint who resides in a twin-towered pink palace with 2,500 disciples.'

'They sound like fun,' said Kate. 'What are they up to now?'

'Oh, they're both really happy; Astrid is running personal development workshops from her base in Hong Kong, returning to Osho's five-star spiritual spa in Pune for Tantra workshops every Christmas, and Cartier has given up the corporate life to become a fully qualified yoga teacher and manage an art gallery in Beijing. She's so smart – I can just imagine her, her long dark hair tucked behind her tiny ears, her glasses perched on the end of her nose as she pores over an invaluable Tibetan Thangka, knowledgeably describing the complex elements of Buddhist cosmology to the customer standing beside her, a handsome man who breathes in her heavenly scent as he plucks up the courage to ask her out for dinner...'

Kate laughed the big fat laugh I'd already come to love, a laugh so much bigger than her body that it always took me by surprise. Thus encouraged I described my brush with the 'liberated while living' yoga tribe at Jivamukti in New York, the Park Avenue Princesses of Exhale and the scriptwriters of LA.

'There's an LA branch of my family,' admitted Kate, 'and I have thought about going out there to live but I don't think Will would find it very easy to transfer his skills and anyway, I think I'd prefer to be the founding member of the Yoga Ibiza tribe – I can see us now – we're a mellow bunch, practising in the late afternoon sun on a deck above the beach, listening to the sound of the sea and a Café Del Mar soundtrack as the sun casts its long rays over our bodies.'

Now *that* was a tribe to join.

Whatever the exact composition of the individual yoga tribes the great thing, we agreed, was that all tribes are members of a 'matocracy', a People's Republic of Yoga in which we are all equal.

'Think about it,' said Kate excitedly, 'we leave our attachment to houses and designer shoes outside the door of the yoga studio and in that space we're content to walk in bare feet, to occupy mats of a broadly uniform size, to be united by nothing more than our breath.'

'Of course that's the theory but in reality status, power and sheer competitiveness do crash through the yoga studio doors,' I reminded Kate. 'There are teachers with rock-star entourages, students who are apparently willing to spend £200 on a Marc Jacobs yoga mat bag and students who spend their whole time engaged in unofficial "who's got the best body?" contests. When I was in Mysore I saw lots of poolside swimsuit contests where a one per cent gain in Body Mass Index could lose a yoga girl the game.'

But, as I made my way home, I had a feeling that if the People's Republic of Yoga could happen anywhere it could happen here in Beccles – Kate was notably disinterested in entourages, and there was a distinct absence of body contests, despite the presence of an outdoor pool just up the road – I couldn't imagine any of us asking 'does my *Uddiyana Bandha* look big in this?' For one thing we all wore too many layers of clothing.

The following week I went to Kiki's class again. I was glad to get out of the house; David had man flu and had come up to the house so I could be his nurse/slave for a week. His recovery was a slow one and he was driving me mad with his cravings – today it had been dim sum soup. We'd gone to all three Chinese restaurants in Beccles and they'd all been closed – clearly there wasn't much demand for Chinese on a Tuesday lunchtime. We ended up in Tesco faced with a choice between Chinese Curry Pot Noodle and a packet of miso soup. The Pot Noodle was soon rejected and yours truly made an approximation of dim sum using the packet miso, chillies (lots of chillies), tofu and pak choi. He got all huffy at being left alone but I swear it was for his own good – I'd have cheerfully murdered him if I'd had to endure another night of extra-virulent man flu.

Once again Kiki's class was a juicy affair, she walked amongst us exhorting us to use 'breath and *bandhas*' as the temperature rose to match the colour of her yoga workwear. She demonstrated postures with ease and grace and her adjustments were masterful – I watched as she pulled the most stubborn of bodies into a pretzel-like shape and my *Urdhva Dhanurasana,* a strong backbend, opened significantly when she gently coaxed my shoulders towards the back of the room, though such was the intensity of the stretch I did wonder if this might be my Corpse Pose.

Not only was she technically sound, she also had a sense of humour; 'Doesn't my foot feel like a car jack under your bum?' she said as she leveraged my left hip upwards till it was level with the right. The intense front body stretch and flat stomach of *Purvottanasana* or Reclining Plank, was rechristened *Spanksasana* in honour of the tummy control pants. 'Let's do *Dhanurasana*,' she'd say with the enthusiasm of a child. 'Now ladies, put your hands back to your bra strap and men, well just imagine you're wearing a bra and put your hands there.'

Not surprisingly I finished the class in good humour and Kiki emerged from behind the yoga screen as a forties film-noir heroine complete with black fake fur coat belted at the waist and a fedora hat that cast an alluring shadow across her face. It was becoming clear that Kiki was never knowingly underdressed. We walked, her in scarlet heels and me in my now clean black boots, through Norwich's medieval streets to Baba Ghanoush. The waitress lit the candle between us, took our order and we got down to business over the obligatory glass of Pinot Grigio.

I was soon admitting to feeling a bit maudlin about my chances of pregnancy, which would probably be halved by the glass of Pinot Grigio I was about to drink. In truth life in the country was increasing my desire for children. After years of denial – never even allowing myself the possibility of motherhood until I met David – now I saw children everywhere, and I was uncovering some long-buried maternal instincts; I even began to think that I might be quite good at it.

'I just wish I'd got on with it sooner,' I said, 'it seems as if every woman of my age has teenage children, there's you, my friends Poppy and Gabriele... David and I went to a barbecue in the summer and I saw this glamorous forty-something woman channelling Eva Longoria Parker as she weaved her way across the lawn in vertiginous heels and white skinny jeans, clutching a bottle of champagne. "Surely she doesn't have children," I thought to myself, but yes, of course she did – two teenage boys as good-looking as their mother trailed unwillingly behind her.'

'I'm sure she—'

'Then, at the same party, there was this woman called Chatty, I mean what kind of a name is that?' I asked indignantly, conscious that I might be sounding bitter. 'She was in her mid-forties, a chisel-faced woman with a less than relaxed manner, and even she'd managed to produce a lush fifteen-year-old who captivated all the men's attention with a pair of milky white bosoms which kept threatening to spill out of her tiny tank top.'

I mused on my life choices while Kiki struggled to get a word in edgeways. 'Why did I decide to start my career at the age of nine?' I asked, explaining that I'd been born a working girl; that there'd been no time for playing with dolls or miniature prams. 'Why didn't I settle down to a life of play dates over glasses of gin and tonic with Eva Longoria Parker and Chatty?'

'Because you're not that kind of girl,' suggested Kiki gently, 'you're an independent woman, you—'

'You know, David is so relaxed about our prospects,' I said, interrupting her again, conscious that I might've had one glass too many. 'He says to me, "Don't worry, Babe – it'll just happen"; he seems to think that if it doesn't happen then it doesn't matter, he says that we have so much in our lives not having children isn't an issue, but I'm less certain – both of our prospects and of it not being an issue.'

'I totally understand, Lucy,' said Kiki, pouring me a glass of water. 'I'm just thinking about what else you should try. Have you looked at *Luna Yoga* – the book that Kate gave you – yet?'

'You mean "Loony Yoga"?' I said miserably. 'It wasn't really my thing, Kiki; all those pelvic rolls, all that stomping around with outstretched arms, all the Heavenly Energy, Chopping Wood and Harvest Dances – it made me feel a bit mad, and anyway it was hard to do the exercises with decorators in the house.'

Kiki agreed readily that this might be something of a deal breaker and we moved on to her love life, which, I was quickly learning, was tumultuous. Clearly a very bright girl who'd achieved no small measure of academic success – she might have a Masters, a work-in-progress PhD, and a part-time university lecturer position – but she'd had considerably less success in love.

'Perhaps the surfer will work out,' I said, trying to be positive.

'Oh, I don't expect there's any long-term future in it,' she said sadly, ordering another glass of wine for both of us. 'He's young, he lives in Devon and I'm just so busy with raising my son, writing my PhD and all my yoga classes – they really do have to be my priority right now.'

'It must be so tough raising children single-handedly,' I said sympathetically. 'How long have you been on your own?'

'I split up with my husband five years ago,' she said, sighing. 'Then there was the man I thought you were with in Mysore, then some single time, and then there was Prawn Man – we split up in January.'

'Prawn Man?'

'Yes, I was with him for a year, but I should've left sooner – he was horrible to me – really emotionally abusive…'

'In what way did he abuse you?' I asked, shocked.

'Loads – but the best was when he couldn't cope with me throwing up after a dodgy prawn curry in Stoke Newington. There was I riding the china bus and needing a good back rub and for him to hold my hair out of my face and all he could do was tell me to go to my mother's house and throw up there.'

'I hope that you chucked him as soon as you'd finished chucking up,' I said, sounding rather stern.

'Oh yes,' said Kiki quickly, 'but I still miss him.'

I concentrated on my roast pepper salad for a moment; to my mind she was unfathomably heartbroken by this man.

'And what's happened since January?' I asked.

'Well, now there's the surfer – God knows how long that will last, I think it's just a fling – but I had a couple of "interesting" dates after Prawn Man. One was with a man whose first wife had died but that ended with us weeping into our Pinot Grigio together, the other one was going really well until he let slip that his parents had been Nazis in Germany…'

'That's awful but he's not responsible for his parents – it's not necessarily a reason to reject—'

'I'm Jewish,' interrupted Kiki, draining her glass.

There was a moment of silence in which I polished off the remains of my Pinot Grigio, and then we both burst out laughing.

9

'A super-high concentrate of antifreeze'

The clocks went back and the town said a sad goodbye to the last brave Hoseasons holidaymakers as they surrendered the keys to their motor cruiser, drank down the dregs of their thermos and packed up their cagoules. There were upsides to this desertion; the average speed on the roads almost doubled when the caravans left and we no longer needed to book a restaurant table a month in advance, but a chill had descended that was hard to shift. The harvest left the fields with hard furrowed ridges, the rich brown earth merging with the spiky brown hedges. I returned from my walks in the leaf-poor, fungi-rich woods with cold cheeks and a red nose. Taking a cup of tea out to Bill, our sixty-year-old born-and-bred-in-Norfolk gardener, became an ordeal as the easterly wind blew in from the Atlantic. 'Yew fare frawn today? Got to harden yew up, gerl,' he said, laughing at my shivering. I didn't know how he could be out there for hours on end in the 'smeurie' as he called it – actually I did, the man had the constitution of an ox and a rather un-ox-like penchant for Morrison's just-baked jam doughnuts. He could easily consume five in the time it took him to weed one of our flowerbeds. They were sold in packs of six so I was sometimes a beneficiary – examining the doughnut to body-weight ratio my one to his five was about right.

One day, watching the ewes being clipped, and hearing that the dairy cows were calving again I realised that nature was entering a new cycle and I patently wasn't. Even Bill was at it – his wife, twenty years younger than him, had just given birth to a little boy. 'We hadn't planned it, I've already got grown-up children – she just looked at me and she fell pregnant,' he told me proudly, licking the sugar off his huge fingers, 'and she's forty-two – can you believe it, sprogging at her age? That's a proper clodhopper's genes fer yew.'

And then my stepsister gave birth, aged thirty-eight, to Jessica. Mum and Oliver flew down to Exeter to see her, the girl who would surf before she could walk, and returned pronouncing Jo 'an excellent mother'. Victoria, my other stepsister, fell immediately in love with her niece and every-one speculated when she herself would 'fall'. I noticed that no one speculated about me.

With a sinking feeling I realised that I'd been trying to get pregnant for a year now; now I would be classed as officially 'infertile' – a word that made me feel like an old hag – and officially worried. The more time I spent in the country the more I wanted a child and the further away it seemed to be getting. A concerned Kiki pointed me in the direction of a community website for infertile women that a friend of hers had found useful. I spent a toe-curling hour scrolling through women's profiles – an initially bewilder-ing list of shorthanded fertility tests, results, and medications that, once translated, revealed a depressing litany of failed attempts:

Me 25, DH 28
TTC 6 years
2 early MC 05
6x Clomid 05
1IVF 10 eggs, BFN
2 & 3 nat FET, 2 x chem. Pg
4 IVF 19 eggs, 5 grade 1 BFN
5 IVF 16 eggs, 6 grade 1 BFN
6 IVF 30 eggs, 14 embies, 2 exp blastocysts, 2AA,
    2BB BFN
Why? Why? Why?

Why? Why? Why? Indeed. Some Harvard research had found that women being treated for infertility could develop the same level of anxiety as cancer patients. I wasn't surprised. I wondered if the women behind the numbers felt they'd lost themselves. And at what point? To paraphrase Peggy Orenstein's *Waiting for Daisy*, the story of her quest to have a baby, the roads called Desire and Denial seemed to have merged at a place called Obsession. I was clear – I didn't want to get anywhere near this place. I talked it through with David and we agreed we needed to consult the experts; we needed facts, we needed to find out why I wasn't getting pregnant.

Well past my sell-by date for any help from the NHS, a fact that angered me as a tax-paying citizen, I did some research on fertility clinics, which largely involved speaking to Gabriele who proved to be a mine of information on the subject, largely due to the experiences of the mums she'd met through her own children. The word at the school gates was that Dr Marie Wren was the main woman.

'She's fabled amongst older women who've had trouble getting pregnant,' said Gabriele. 'They tell me that she's one of the best and most sympathetic fertility experts in the country.'

We arrived at the Lister hospital, a vast building over-looking the Thames, on a bright sunny Monday morning. We eventually found the fertility clinic hidden away on a half floor, which gave it a disconcertingly furtive air. David went off to give his sample and I went for an ultrasound, return-ing to sit nervously in the packed waiting room – it was full of couples the same age as, or a bit younger than, us. I smiled weakly at some of the other women but it was clear that in this environment eye contact was forbidden and I settled into hiding behind a copy of the *Daily Telegraph* – as the biggest broadsheet it offered the most coverage. David returned with tales of a plastic beaker, a vinyl daybed and a television that didn't show the usual channels – we giggled together – mission accomplished.

Dr Wren came to collect us and we followed her up the corridor, past a woman sobbing in the arms of her man. I tried not to feel rattled, focusing instead on keeping our doctor in my sights: an attractive blonde evoking Stevie Nicks in a tiered skirt and wafting pale blue bell-sleeved shirt accessorised with lots of beads.

We sat in her warm office high above Chelsea Embank-ment and I explained that we'd been trying for a year, and that although we had wanted to do things the natural way we were now prepared to consider IVF as we were conscious that time was running out. Dr Wren sat behind her huge antique desk and listened sympathetically, occasionally adjust-ing her glasses, making notes, hunting for information in the large pile of papers before, beside and behind her. She reviewed the results of my ultrasound and David's sperm test.

'David's results are not very good,' she said slowly, squinting at the piece of paper displaying a set of numbers only she could interpret.

Now this was an unexpected scenario – I'd never thought it might be David's 'problem'.

'When did you last have sex?' she asked, looking up over her glasses.

'Last night,' said David. 'I've just got back from a friend's stag weekend in Ibiza and we've been making up for lost time.'

'Oh,' she said, crumpling up the piece of paper detailing the results. 'That probably explains it – you're supposed to abstain from sex for three days before you take the test. Didn't anyone tell you?'

No they didn't.

'And Lucy, your ultrasound is hard to read – I can see five follicles on one ovary but the other side is blurred by an ovarian cyst, and you have a polyp. I suggest that we conduct a "gynaecological MOT": give you a Laparoscopy and Hysteroscopy, remove the cyst and the polyp, which may be getting in the way of conception, and check your Fallopian tubes. Let's repeat David's sperm test and get day three FSH and oestrogen readings for you Lucy – that will tell us about your eggs...'

'What's FSH?' I asked.

'Follicle Stimulating Hormone is the main hormone involved in producing eggs,' explained Dr Wren, adjusting her glasses. 'The higher the number of egg follicles, and the better their quality, the less FSH needs to be produced to get the follicle production started. So, the lower the level of

FSH the better – ten or under is good.' She got up and opened the door for us. 'I'll see you both again in a month when we have more information.'

We left feeling optimistic and emerged into the sunshine congratulating ourselves, and Gabriele, on finding Dr Wren – she was 'so straightforward', 'so experienced' and 'so knowledgeable'. We walked back to the car busily assuring ourselves that the sperm test would be fine next time round, that five follicles would probably be enough and that a gynaecological MOT was an excellent idea. More than anything these things felt like progress and, after months of waiting for something to happen, progress felt good.

I went back to Norfolk to await my appointment with the surgeon's knife. Two days before I was due for the gynaecological MOT the Met Office issued a storm surge warning for the East Anglia coast. Force eight winds were predicted to push high tide water south into the narrow waters around Great Yarmouth, Lowestoft and down into Suffolk, creating three-metre-high surges on the morning of 9 November. The Norfolk and Suffolk Gold Command, the Fire and Rescue National Flood Support Centre and the cabinet met to discuss strategy. This was a big deal.

Kate and I had planned to spend a restorative evening at The Locks Inn in Geldeston – a picturesque pub on the River Waveney. I rang to ask them whether, given the weather, they were open.

'It depends what car you drive,' the landlady replied.

'That's a bit of a personal question – I don't think you should stop me coming if I don't drive a particular car,' I said hotly.

'It's not us – it's the water that says so. Tractors and four by fours only, I'm afraid – the road is already flooded.'

I looked at Kate. Neither of us had a spare tractor to hand.

'Another time, then,' I said.

'Unless you have a boat?' suggested the Locks Inn landlady helpfully.

We didn't have one of those either.

It was a night to stay in.

I made us toad in the hole, we needed comfort food, and we sat in front of the roaring woodburner transfixed by *News 24*, watching in morbid fascination as camera crews accosted the people of Great Yarmouth and Lowestoft.

'What preparations are you making for tonight?' asked the BBC reporter dressed in a billowing windcheater.

'We've got a few sandbags from my brother-in-law,' said a large lady with hoop earrings filling out the doorway of her house. 'We're lucky really because he's a brickie – my neighbour says the council have run out.'

'And we've moved the big telly upstairs to our mam's bedroom,' her spiky-haired, khaki-clad son piped up.

'Along with the five kids,' she continued, folding her arms and smiling with that special brand of grit and humour that the English do so well in times of adversity.

The Environment Agency's representative spoke of potential 'extreme danger to people and property'. A rest area for homeless evacuees had been established in Beccles, so-called 'spotters' had been posted at strategic vantage points to monitor the rising water, the local radio stations were broadcasting through the night.

Kate began to worry about whether she would be able

to get back to Harleston without a boat and left early – swept home by the drenching driving rain.

I stayed up listening to local radio most of the night – should I ring the Dom and offer up our house as a sanctuary for evacuees – a safe house in a storm? I could make piping hot sugared tea and dispense McVities digestive biscuits, organise a spirits lifting game of Monopoly or Spilikins.

In the end it came to little. When I woke up at eight – having finally fallen asleep at five – the crisis in Great Yarmouth and Lowestoft had already been averted. The tidal surge hadn't coincided with the high tide and the wind direction had changed – from north-westerly to westerly – so in the words of Norfolk Radio there had been 'no drama'. I listened to the radio all morning but as the tide moved down the coast each town reported only minor problems – a closed road due to flooding, shingle damage at a local bird sanctuary and a buried footpath at Walberswick.

I found out later, during another gathering at Lady Birkie's house, that the Sex Therapist's eighty-year-old mother, a woman who still stands to attention whenever the national anthem is played, was a British Civil Defence volunteer – 'the nation's best defence against Al Qaeda', as the Sex Therapist said. Dressed in a nuclear fall-out suit, set off by sturdy boots and an orange sweatshirt, her team had been in charge of supporting the east Norfolk coast's emergency services. She'd made tea and bacon sandwiches for the local police, manned the BCD's four-by-four ambulances, managed their stash of flashlights, torches, buoyancy aids, and ground to satellite emergency location transmitters. If only we'd known that she was in charge we wouldn't have worried.

*

I wished I'd had the Sex Therapist's mother on hand to make me cups of tea at the Lister but I was Nil by Mouth until the operation. Despite knowledge of this deprivation I'd been looking forward to my day in bed. I was giving up more than a cup of tea – my medical insurance company had refused to cover me for what they claimed was a pre-existing condition so we'd had to find the money to pay for this operation ourselves. I was determined to make the most of it – imagining that, due to the eye-watering cost of the procedure, it would be like travelling first class; there'd be latest-release DVDs, a mountain of magazines and someone interesting in the next bed to chat to. The reality was a little different – I was given a hermetically sealed room of my own and despite its obvious comforts it was quite clearly a hospital room. David left and I suddenly felt very small and alone. Why hadn't I prepared myself for this? A nurse came in and went through a form with me, then she gave me a paper gown and knickers and some long white stockings to prevent deep-vein thrombosis. By the time I was wheeled into theatre at one in the afternoon I'd been without so much as a glass of water for fifteen hours and I felt so dehydrated it was as if I'd downed three bottles of Pinot Grigio the previous night.

I'd also completely underestimated how bad I was going to feel afterwards – I thought that I'd be back on my feet the very next day, but I woke up from the operation feeling terrible – my stomach was swollen like a balloon, I could hardly move and I felt really low, something to do with the anaesthetic, apparently. David came to collect me and sat with me all evening, stroking my fevered brow and administrating four-hourly doses of paracetamol. I retired to bed and a couple of days later I caught the train back to Norfolk to convalesce, spending the next week moving around the house with the ease of a ninety-year-old who'd just had both hips replaced. I'd wanted to keep news of the operation quiet – partly because I thought it would be routine – no worse than a trip to the dentist – but when I didn't turn up at my yoga classes the following week Kiki rang to find out what had happened to me, and soon after that the two Bad Ladies popped round with a bunch of flowers and a large tub of Kiki's chicken soup.

I almost didn't recognise Dr Wren when we saw her again ten days later. She appeared to be in a very different mood – wearing black trousers and a polo neck. I hoped this wasn't a signifier of bad news.

David and I drew our chairs close together and towards her large desk.

Leafing through the reports in front of her she adjusted her turquoise-lined spectacles and crossed her hands under her chin.

'Your Lap and Hys results are fine, Lucy, your Fallopian tubes are healthy, the polyp and a two-centimetre cyst were removed from your ovary and, although I still can't see the number of follicles on the ultrasound scan – because the cyst hasn't fully disappeared yet – everything looks okay.' She studied my hormone results. 'Your oestrogen level is a little elevated but your FSH level of seven is excellent and,' a long pause as she studied another piece of paper, 'David's sperm results are good – much better than last time.'

Thank goodness for that, we can just go back to Norfolk and everything will be fine; I might even be pregnant by Christmas. No festive drinking for me, oh well, a sacrifice worth making. But Dr Wren was saying something else…

'... and yet you are not getting pregnant. The most likely explanation is age – when a woman reaches her forties we have to recognise that we're working with older eggs, and I am afraid that their quality declines over time. So, the question is what we do next.'

She spooled through some numbers on her computer. There was another long pause.

She turned her chair to face me head on and fixed me with her intensely blue eyes.

Something in her manner signified that she had bad news. I wished I could freeze time, have it stand still so that I would never have to hear what was coming next.

'A woman of forty-three or forty-four has a thirteen per cent chance of getting pregnant with IVF, and a seventy per cent chance of miscarriage. So, Lucy,' she said, speaking slowly, 'your net chance of delivering a baby using IVF is around four per cent. I'm really sorry.'

'But I thought the odds would be around twenty-five per cent,' I said, my voice wobbling, 'that's the figure that's always bandied around. I know that the chances of getting pregnant naturally diminish with age but I thought IVF fixed all that.'

'The high miscarriage rate amongst older women is due to the age of the eggs not the age of the womb, old eggs just don't implant or develop so easily,' said Dr Wren softly.

'It's okay, Babe,' said David, moving his chair closer to mine and giving my shoulder a reassuring squeeze.

'But I know of several women who've given birth in their forties, and what about all those older celebrity mums – how can that be?' I asked, my throat tickling, my voice high and tight.

'Yes,' agreed Doctor Wren, 'it's really misleading – lots of those women have received donated eggs from younger women – it significantly increases your chances, up to around twenty-five per cent, because you adopt the biological age of the egg donor. Would you consider that option?'

'I don't know,' I said. My head was all furred up, like the inside of an old kettle.

'Perhaps you might also consider adoption,' suggested Dr Wren.

'We will have a think about it,' I said uncertainly, looking at David whose set jaw suggested that he wouldn't need to think about it for very long. He left the room to put some money in the parking meter. I envied him the fresh air; I was suddenly feeling stiflingly hot.

'Such a shame that male fertility doesn't diminish at the same rate as women's,' mused Dr Wren. 'It creates such pressure on the relationship – I see lots of women who are worried because a man can leave and find a younger woman – but,' she paused, 'David doesn't seem to be like that.'

'No, he's not,' I agreed, choking back tears.

'Maybe it's an Indian thing but he seems very accepting of the situation.'

'He is,' I croaked.

'You're very lucky.'

'I know,' I said, staring at the floor and wiping away a tear. There was another long pause.

'Is there anything I can do to help myself?' I asked, desperate to latch on to something positive, some action I could take. 'I've heard that acupuncture can be very good, and one of my friends saw a nutritionist and got pregnant the next month.'

'Anything that makes you feel better is good,' said Dr Wren kindly. 'This whole process can be very disempowering for women and alternative therapies can help with that.'

David returned and Dr Wren wrapped up. 'As you are having normal cycles, your tubes are normal and David has good sperm your chances of conceiving naturally are probably as good as they are with fertility treatment. If you do still want to pursue treatment then come back and I'd be happy to see you. Have a think about it. Talk it through together. I am always here if you want to discuss it again.'

We thanked her and left, walking slowly up towards Pimlico. I was thankful to be outside, to feel the sun on my face again, but inside I was still numb. David suggested some lunch but I'd totally lost my appetite. We stood on the corner of Ebury Street.

'Don't worry, Babe,' he said, folding me into his arms. 'We'll work something out.'

'Like what?' I asked angrily, breaking away from his embrace. Dr Wren may have been endlessly sympathetic and supportive, but there was no getting away from the numbers; an investment of £5,000 per IVF cycle for a four per cent chance of success was not an attractive proposition.

'Just get clear,' said David, wrapping his arms around me again so I couldn't move, 'it *will* happen. We don't need IVF, egg donation or adoption. I've always known I will have children and together we will.'

David's instincts were generally pretty well founded but I couldn't help wondering if his children would have a different mother.

*

153

I returned to Norfolk, which in the few days I'd been away seemed to have plunged into the depths of winter – Fresh and Fruity was full of cauliflowers, beetroot, swedes, parsnips and leeks. The grass had stopped growing, the cows and calves had moved inside, the nights had drawn in, and I settled down in front of the computer to learn about fertility and the older woman, something I should have done years ago.

I spent most of my time on the Human Fertility and Embryology Authority (HFEA) website which licenses and regulates the fertility industry. I spent hours spooling through their collated statistics. It made for riveting, if disturbing, reading.

The bottom line was that the new reproductive technologies didn't seem to have solved the problem for us older birds; according to their most recent data the average IVF success rate for under thirty-fives was thirty per cent, by forty-three, my age now, the chances had plummeted, as Dr Wren said, to four per cent.

While success rates for under thirty-five-year-olds had doubled in the past fifteen years, there'd been no improvement in success rates for women in their early forties. I seemed to belong to the generation that fertility technology forgot. And even if I got pregnant, as Dr Wren had said, the problems wouldn't stop there. I hoovered up Sylvia Ann Hewlett's 2003 best-seller *Creating a Life*. Here I discovered that while eight per cent of twenty-two-year-olds miscarry, at forty-eight that figure is a staggering eighty-four per cent. If a foetus did manage to take root there was, at forty-five, a one in twenty-six chance of chromosomal abnormalities (at twenty-five the figure was one in 1,250.) Older women were more likely to give birth prematurely, risking low baby weights, and even if the baby got through birth in one piece, there was a significant risk of infant mortality; ten to twenty per cent would die within the first year; beyond that there stretched the threat of physical and mental developmental problems throughout childhood.

Finishing the book I had to acknowledge that I was what you might call a fertility fuck-up. Yes, I was healthy, yes, I looked after myself, yes, I did yoga four times a week, and yes, I was a religious user of Olay Regenerist but no, it made no odds. My ovaries were more than forty years old and no anti-wrinkle cream on earth was going to iron out those shrivelled-up old prunes.

Why hadn't I known all this before? Had I been burying my head in the sand? Had I been afraid to face the truth? It was ironic really – I'd spent two years sharing a house at university with a girl with a penchant for miniskirts and heels, and a father called Dr Robert Edwards. He, along with Dr Patrick Steptoe, was responsible for Louise Brown, the world's first test-tube baby. I'd been in such close proximity to the font of all knowledge and I'd never chosen to ask any questions. I guess that at eighteen fertility issues were non-issues.

I could take some comfort in the fact that I wasn't the only one who didn't know the facts – in Sylvia Ann Hewlett's large-scale research a massive eighty-nine per cent of young high-achieving women believed they would be able to get pregnant well into their forties. It wasn't surprising really – we read books that promised to reveal 'how to get pregnant into your forties and fifties with just a few tweaks to diet and lifestyle'. Every time we picked up a paper we learned of another mother who'd succeeded in extending her fertility shelf life. The celebrity roll call of older mothers exuded easy glamour – Cheryl Tiegs may have used a surrogate mother but the surrogate used fifty-two-year-old Cheryl's own eggs, Jane Seymour and Iman both had children at forty-four, Mimi Rogers was forty-five, Susan Sarandon forty-six, Holly Hunter forty-seven. Each headline, each celebrity, had seemingly extended our projected fertility another five years, confirming that yes, we could put it off until well into our forties.

I was feeling angry. These headlines should carry a government health warning for lulling a generation of women into a false sense of security. I didn't begrudge these celebrities their 'baby joy' headlines, I just wished that those who'd used donor eggs had admitted to using them, done their bit to educate women that getting pregnant in their forties was not likely to be as easy as airbrushing out their wrinkles for the glossy magazine 'baby joy' feature.

The following Wednesday I went to Kate's class. Although it did something to dissipate my anger I found myself at the end of class, still quite desperate for a drink. Kate was amenable and disappeared into the tiny kitchen at the back of the Quaker Meeting House, metamorphosing in moments from yoga chick to Ibiza babe, complete with miniskirt, oversized black jumper, taupe tights, and biker boots. Walking the couple of hundred yards from the Meeting House to The Swan House was a satisfying experience – heads swivelled as she passed by, conversation stopped.

We took our drinks to what I'd come to regard as our sofa by the fire and ordered a couple of glasses of Rioja and some treacle tart to share. I got down to business straight away – I was on a one-woman mission to alert my younger friends to the facts of fertility, beginning with Kate, aged thirty-one.

'Did you know that your fertility has already peaked?' I asked her.

'No, I had no idea,' she said, taking a gulp of Rioja.

'Did you know that by the age of thirty it's dropped twenty per cent, that by the time you are thirty-five it will be down by fifty per cent, and by forty, if you're still hanging around on the matter, the figure will be ninety per cent.'

'No, I had no idea,' she repeated. 'I knew it went down a bit but I didn't realise by how much.'

'Well, maybe you and Will should talk about it,' I suggested, firmly.

'We *have* talked about it but we just aren't ready yet,' she said, just as firmly.

'You know, Kate, I thought I had all the time in the world – I thought that because I was used to having choices, to determining my own destiny, that I could choose to have a baby when I wanted to – when I met the man of my dreams – you, on the other hand, are in the lucky position of having a husband who loves you – why not get started?'

'I'd rather not force it on us at this stage – we don't want to be guided by time, we want to be guided by when it's right.'

'Wake up!' I said, suddenly conscious that I might be shouting at my easy-going, mild-mannered friend. 'This is one area in which you have no choice. None! You are a smart woman – use your brain – you are fertile now, but you might not be in five years' time.'

'I know, Lucy, and I understand that you're upset – it's just that—'

I cut her off. 'Kate,' I said, getting frustrated, 'you can resuscitate your career in yoga but you can't resuscitate your ovaries.'

There was a silence; we sipped our Rioja.

'Do you have a five-year plan?' I asked her, a little more gently.

She shook her head, looking nervous.

'Then I suggest that you do a Four Corners Collage – each corner represents an aspect of your life – relationship, home, family, work. I did one the year before I met David – I filled my relationship corner with a man and woman having a pillow fight because I wanted a playful partner, my work corner was a picture of a woman writing, piles of books on her desk, the home corner had a picture of a couple sitting beneath an oak tree in the countryside, my family corner had a bunch of friends dressed in designer outfits inspired by the union jack flag. And guess what,' I said triumphantly, 'I got everything I wanted.' I stared into my glass of Rioja. 'Well, almost everything,' realising for the first time that the collage contained no pictures of children – I really had cut myself off from that possibility, until I met David.

'That's a good idea, Lucy,' agreed Kate. 'I do believe that if we are clear about what we want it will manifest itself.'

'Exactly,' I agreed, driving the conversation towards my stated goal – I was taking no prisoners. 'You need to ask yourself: "What will it take for me to be happy now? In two years' time? In five years' time?" Get some magazines and start tearing out pictures that appeal to you, that say something about where you want to be – get clear, because one thing's for sure

– if you don't manage your life it will manage you.'

Kate looked a bit shell-shocked but I wished that someone had had this conversation with me when I was her age.

'There is one other thing you should consider if you want to extend your fertility,' I suggested.

'What's that?' asked Kate carefully.

'Freezing your eggs – so you can have a so-called "ice baby" later, when you're ready. The success rates are about half as good as using fresh eggs – that's why it's not recommended for women in their forties but for women under thirty-five it's better than nothing, and the techniques are improving all the time. Sometimes the eggs don't survive the freezing process and there is a danger ice crystals can form which might damage the genetic material in the egg but I read about a new technique called EVES – it's early days so there isn't that much data yet, we're only talking about around 150 pregnancies in total around the world – but it's getting an eighty-five per cent egg fertilisation success rate, which is better than conventional freezing methods. In conventional freezing the temperature goes down by less than a degree per minute, whereas EVES uses a flash-freezing methodology with a super-high concentrate of antifreeze to reduce that risk.'

'Antifreeze?' asked Kate quizzically. 'Are you sure?' She looked concerned.

'Yes, antifreeze,' I said confidently; I'd done my research. 'It drops the temperature much faster – something like 23,000 degrees centigrade per minute – making it 70,000 times faster than the standard method.'

I could see that Kate remained unconvinced but she did agree to do her Four Corner Collage. I left happy, I'm not

sure she did but I tried not to let it worry me – reasoning
that being an inconsiderate harridan, riding roughshod over
a friend's sensitivities, was perfectly okay if I saved her from
what looked to be my likely fate.

10

'If I needed a soulful cruise I'd head to East Runton'

I channelled my anger and frustration over the four per cent news into preparing for our first Christmas in the farmhouse. I ordered a huge turkey from the local butcher and dozens of mince pies from Goulborn's, my favourite stall at the Beccles farmers' market. We watched Terry Molloy, who played *Doctor Who*'s Davros (the cyberkinetic-eyed Dalek creator) and Mike Tucker (*The Archers'* one-eyed milkman with a penchant for *Strictly Strumpy*-style line dancing), turn on Beccles' Christmas lights. (He appeared to have two fully functioning eyes in this role.) We chanced upon the Dom and wandered with him from stall to stall in the pouring rain, getting a priest's-eye view of the world in which everyone says 'hello' and offers you a glass of mulled wine. We went to the children's carol service, revelling in Mary's white fur halo and the four-year-old wise men's Bacofoil headdresses, marvelling at the five-year-olds' brass ensemble and their imposing rendition of 'Jingle Bells', giving some money to the collection for St Benet's twin 'school of peace' in the

Congo. I plucked holly from our bushes to make centre-pieces for the table and sent Christmas hampers full of home-made jam, mince pies (Goulborn's were so much better than my own) and ginger wine to London as promised. We warmed ourselves with logs left by the back door, a present from the local farmer, and we opened the champagne when our painter finished work the Friday before Christmas – a job that had kept him occupied, on and off, since the summer.

Christmas Eve brought my stepsisters to the farmhouse and being around Jessica – now nearly three months old – was bittersweet. She was a robust and pretty child with big blue eyes and an easy smile. I watched Jo, for thirty-eight years a hyperactive overachiever, in her new role as an earth mother – fully secure in herself for the first time in her life. Jessica looked at her with such certainty that Jo became certain of herself; because Jessica knew who Jo was so Jo knew who she was. While Jo had found herself I felt as if I'd almost certainly lost myself as a mother. I read that having children is like watching your heart being carried around in someone else. Would my heart only ever live inside of me?

I didn't want to share these thoughts with anyone, least of all myself, so I hid in the kitchen cooking a Christmas feast and lecturing my youngest stepsister, thirty-six-year-old Victoria, on the daily deterioration in her fertility. I'd suggested that she return to London and get her eggs on ice before she unpacked her suitcase. 'You don't have a minute to spare, you know – most fertility clinics cut off their egg freezing programmes at thirty-seven.' Victoria said little, skilfully deflecting the conversation back to the marvels of Jo and Jessica.

I'd been limited to three glasses of Pinot Grigio per week for six months and, bar the odd night out with Kiki and Kate, I'd managed to stick to it, but now, fuelled by the feeling that it probably didn't matter anymore, I knocked back three glasses a night. I was officially a Bad Lady now and I behaved appropriately. I recovered from my hangovers with bracing walks. The local farmer had been busy to the last; ploughing, spreading slurry and calving; now the fields lay uncharacteristically silent, bar the pheasants which were everywhere; we watched them waddling as fast as they could along the track ahead of us, their fat bodies wobbling from side to side, desperate to get out of our way but somehow unwilling to take flight, eventually disappearing into the woods where they'd lose themselves in rough tangles of brambles and ivy. Our walks were often peppered by the sound of shooting, and the pheasants weren't the only ones worried. We wondered if we might end up in the Sheriff's game keep – our necks sandwiched between two nails, our heads lolling off to one side.

We'd come home to find the shoot's booty hanging from the back door in plastic bags – thank goodness they weren't in their natural state – the birds were so free of feathers and so neatly wrapped in cling film that, if I didn't know better, I'd think the Sheriff had bought them in Tesco.

I was lucky that my urge to parent found some outlet that Christmas – in the form of a chocolate brown cat that arrived on the windowsill with a very strong sense of entitlement. Seduced by the smell of a Christmas feast in the making, the cat was absolutely desperate to come into the house. She tried every trick in the book but we were worried that she might be the treasured darling of a local family who'd gone away for the holidays and would return to look for it, so we banished her to an old bean bag in the shed.

I think David admired her tenacity, hanging on despite the gruelling cold. What he didn't know was that I fed her turkey scraps when he wasn't looking, and when they ran out I added Whiskas to the shopping basket. Eventually, after a week, he softened and even began to worry that she might be depressed (who wouldn't be living in a shed, especially at Christmas?) Seeing her purring in my arms he consented to let her stay – as long as the vet gave her a clean bill of health.

As soon as the vet reopened after Christmas I popped her in a cardboard box, made a hole in the top for air, sealed the box with four metres of brown tape and jumped in the car. Like Houdini she broke out in less than ten seconds and after a precarious spell on my shoulder assumed a much safer driving position – sitting in my lap with her paws on the steering wheel, staring attentively through the windscreen.

I struggled through the surgery door with the cat, back by now in its cardboard box, and took my place amongst dogs who sat silently in varying degrees of misery wearing plastic cones and bandages while the cats yowled inside an assortment of pink, tartan and wickerwork carriers. My cat yowled the loudest, a high-pitched cry that threatened to become a scream at any moment. I was relieved when it was our turn; like a mother with a misbehaving child I was starting to feel embarrassed.

Emma the vet, a capable young woman dressed in green scrubs, lifted the cat on to the examining table and without further ado lifted the tail.

'She's really pretty,' said Emma, looking thoughtfully at her arsehole.

We laughed.

'Really pretty,' she repeated, firmly pulling down the cat's tail and patting it on the back.

My chest swelled with pride.

Now that I knew for sure it was a she I wondered if the bloating I'd noticed was a pregnancy but Emma said not. There was a bit of me that was disappointed – though it would've been hard to know what to do with six kittens I'd have found it auspicious that a pregnant cat had chosen to take shelter with me, a person wanting to be pregnant. The vet gave her a preventative anti-worm course; she thought that had caused the bloating, cheerfully informing me that I'd 'see the worms in a day or two if she has them'.

I wanted to understand why she might've left home. Emma told me that 'cats don't stray unless there's a change of circumstance, say a new baby or dog. They rarely travel more than a mile in any circumstance, unless they've been dumped.' We thought it unlikely that anyone would want to dump such a pretty cat, so perhaps she'd moved on because a baby had taken her place. It would be ironic if I got pregnant and she felt she had to leave again. Still, I thought grimly, that was looking pretty unlikely – they say cats have a sixth sense, can receive information on an astral plane, she probably already knew that the chances of her being turfed out were only four per cent.

I explained that I'd registered her with the local missing cats' society, put her on the Lost and Found list and knocked on the door of all our neighbours.

'Then you've done everything you can,' said Emma

briskly. 'She doesn't have an ownership chip and she's in good health – I'd say give it another week or two and then she's yours.'

In the mood to celebrate I blew my weekly shopping budget on a bag of vet-recommended food, a book on cat care, a litter tray, a food bowl, a fluffy yellow tail on a stick, a catnip mouse and four pink ping pong balls.

The cat was asleep when I got home. I sat down and read *The Cat Bible* cover to cover. It said I should play with her for at least five minutes every few hours. The cat remained asleep. I had to wait six hours for her to wake up – I paced up and down like an anxious father awaiting the birth of his baby. When she woke up she was hungry, then thirsty. Finally the moment came.

She backed away from the yellow tail, sniffed the catnip mouse disdainfully, pushed the ping pong balls out of her way and went back to sleep.

'What shall we call her?' I asked David. 'I was thinking of Bungles – an amalgam of Beccles and Bungay – because we don't know where she is from. Clever isn't it? What do you think?'

'Billa,' said David firmly.

'Billa?'

'Billa is Urdu for cat.'

I watched as Billa, who'd ignored me completely when I called her Bungles, woke up, swivelled her head 180 degrees at the sound of her new name and trotted over to David. She jumped on the sofa and together they fell asleep.

David and I decided that we should bring in what would be our first full year in the farmhouse with a little dinner party.

We invited The Bad Ladies of Norfolk and their partners, and hoped that the London Cappuccino Gurus would join us too but it was not to be; Poppy was busy 'researching' the Balinese yoga scene as inspiration for her boutique yoga centre, Gabriele was in France with her in-laws, and Andrea had a hot date with a recently single Greenpeace lawyer she'd met through her company.

David and I spent four painstaking hours in the kitchen making an Indian feast. We'd been inspired by a recent visit from his sister Cynthia, the first Indian to be awarded a Cordon Bleu Grand Diploma. Her CV read like a Who's Who of fashionable London; she'd been Head Chef at Armani, she'd worked at the River Café, Nicole Farhi, Liberty, Tate Modern and The Sugar Club. Inspired as a child by their Goan chef in Karachi and her mother, whose secret ingredient was 'the two handfuls of love' she added to each dish before serving, Cynthia was happy to pass her knowledge on, teaching me how to make Mangalorean Prawn Curry, a recipe passed down from her great-grandmother. We narrowly avoided disaster when David, in his infinite wisdom, put an extra chilli in the curry – it took the roof of his mouth off and I had to ring Cynthia to discuss resuscitation procedures (for the curry. David's well-being was less important to me at this stage). It quickly assumed a new guise – prawn and potato curry – it wasn't too bad but I sincerely hoped that great-grandma in the sky wasn't watching us.

It was our first-ever dinner party for friends in our just finished dining room, which we'd decorated with Farrow & Ball 'Eating Room Red' on Poppy's recommendation – 'Think about food colours, guys,' she told us, 'that's what works.' She was right, the room looked grand and as David and I took either end of our newly acquired dining table I looked around me with pride. We had Kiki and her surfer, Kate and Will and Billa, and everyone, bar the cat, had made an effort. Even the men were wearing clean T-shirts. In a rare departure from my haute gap-year uniform I was in a black lace dress with opaque tights and black ankle boots, Kate had crimped her hair and come as a seventies girl straight out of the fashion pages of *Jackie* – wearing a long white maxi dress, feather eyelashes and white wedges – and Kiki had really pushed the boat out this time, arriving in a strapless fifties prom gown and matching black and emerald-green heels.

The wine flowed, the fire roared, and we settled in for the night – a night in which we learned all about the correct construction of hedgerows from conservationist Will, and surfing off the Norfolk coast from Kiki's laconic fella.

'How does it compare to Devon?' asked David, turning his tweed cap round in the style of Samuel L. Jackson.

'No comparison, mate,' said the surfer definitively. 'Saunton is the best longboard wave in the UK – it's totally epic. Round here? Well, Gorleston's only worth it when there's a big north swell and everything else has been blown out, when it's firing Walcott has the best tidal rip on the east coast – it's great for sucky waves...' he paused, leaning back in his chair and staring at a faraway spot beyond the ceiling, '... but if I needed a soulful cruise I'd head to East Runton, it's a magic channel on dawn patrol...'

These elemental tales put us in a reflective mood – we watched the cat playing with the triangles of light dancing off our recently purchased chandelier, and allowed ourselves to slide slowly down our chairs and into the soft blur of bonhomie. Eventually the men retired to the sitting room, where David had set up his newly acquired pool table, leaving us Bad Ladies to make our New Year's resolutions.

Kate had an announcement to make. 'We're thinking about selling the house and moving to Ibiza.'

There was a silence much like the one I'd experienced when I'd told The Cappuccino Gurus I was moving to Norfolk.

'When we went there for a holiday last summer we met a group of environmental activists who were clearing up the beach,' explained Kate. 'We got talking to them and went to see their farm. It's an amazing place – it's all very rustic – powered by wind and sun energy, and they recycle all their water. We're thinking of joining them.'

'Permanently?'

'Probably. It would be a way for us to put something back – we've been going to the island as tourists for years and we didn't realise the environmental damage we were doing.'

'What would you do there?'

'Well, Will would help them use their land more effectively – grow vegetables, erect polytunnels, help them get an organic accreditation, that sort of thing. I could help look after the children in the family house, and of course I would teach yoga to the commune, they were really into the idea.'

'It sounds amazing, Kate,' I said, feeling like one of The Cappuccino Gurus on the receiving end of my Norfolk news. Part of me was happy to see her so excited, and admired her idealism, but the other part of me worried about her setting off into the unknown. 'How far down the line are you with this?'

'Oh, nothing is decided yet – I did that Four Corners Collage, Lucy, and it was brilliant – I realised that I didn't want to waste any more time doing admin for a big corporate – I just want to teach yoga and for us to be entirely self-sufficient – so we're looking at some of the ways in which we might be able to make it happen.'

Kate agreed to keep us posted on developments and I tried to focus my thoughts in a positive direction – on the joy of making a difference to Kate's life rather than the downside – losing a new friend, and my Wednesday night yoga class. I was somewhat unsuccessful.

Kiki had received unwelcome news that she needed to share: she had heard that Prawn Man was taking off for six months of caravanning round Europe with his new thirty-year-old bird. I think that her sadness over this loser remained a mystery to us all.

'Do you want to spend six months travelling aimlessly around Europe?' I asked.

'No,' came the reply, her head hanging.

'Do you want to live in a caravan for six months?'

'No.'

'And do you want to be with Prawn Man anymore?'

'No.'

'So why are you so upset?' I asked, uncomprehending.

'I'm sorry,' replied Kiki mournfully, 'it's just that it's his birthday today and I suppose I'm still holding a candle for him.'

'Kiki,' I said gently, 'there is a man in the next room who has come here all the way from Devon just to be with you. Aren't you interested in him?'

'Yes, but I know it's just a fling,' said Kiki miserably. 'I was in love with Prawn Man – we were planning our future together and I'm having real trouble moving on – we were together for a while, and of course there were lots of good times...'

'Isn't it time that you moved on, darling?' Kate suggested gently. 'It's been a year now. You've got so much going for you – your PhD, your classes, your workshops, your tango...'

'You're right,' she said firmly. 'I am going to spend January on a detox – no more skinny lattes, no more Pinot Grigio and no more thinking about toxic men – I will dedicate January to orange juice, yoga, my PhD and having fun with my soulful cruiser.'

'I'll drink to that,' said Kate and I in unison, draining our glasses.

'So how are you feeling now, Lucy?' asked Kate, offering us some home-made chocolates. 'That news of yours was so devastating – and such a surprise...'

'To all of us,' said Kiki, squeezing my hand.

'I've had some time to think about it – to be honest I was pretty angry and I just haven't been sure what to do with myself. I thought about going back to London, putting the whole experience behind me, forgetting my dream, but ladies,' I refilled everyone's glasses, '*this* Bad Lady ain't taking it lying down. I *am* going to beat the odds. The statistics may say four per cent but they are just statistics. I am not a number, I am a human being.'

'Cheers to that, Bad Lady,' said Kiki, lifting her glass to me.

'What does David say?' asked Kate softly.

'He's delighted; he says, "Just get clear, Babe, it will happen".'

And so my New Year's resolution was hatched. 'I hereby

open myself to the possibility of getting pregnant,' I announced, popping another chocolate in my mouth. 'Rather than pumping myself full of IVF drugs in the manner of a battery chicken, being treated as one of "the four per cent" I'm going to submit myself to Norfolk's alternative therapists – the ones specialising in fertility. So, ladies, have you got any recommendations?'

Without further ado The Bad Ladies reached for their mobiles. Five minutes later I was armed with a collection of numbers for Norfolk's finest holistic health gurus.

And so, clutching my scarce and date-stamped eggs to my bosom I got ready to embark on my New Year's quest. Where would the egg and womb race begin? Would I mainline essence of She Oak? Endure the torture of Rolfing? Receive the positive vibrations of a Medicine Man's crystal wand? Would I name the baby Gaia after the New Age therapist who breathed new life into my old eggs? Nothing quite so esoteric – my fertility prescription consisted of a yogic detox, acupuncture, ayurvedic nutrition and Kundalini yoga. Oh, and a tattoo artist.

'He did a tattoo of *Svadhistana chakra* for a friend of mine,' said Kiki, 'it's beautiful and it's a fertility symbol.'

As the friend had apparently gone on to have two children it was certainly worth considering.

I was excited about my prospects. It felt as if there was freedom in this approach, it allowed for hope, the possibility of a miracle.

Although David was very supportive of this new-found positivity he was a little put off by the idea of a big plan. 'Just be relaxed,' he said, trying to persuade me not to do everything in the first week of January. I was not to be persuaded.

11

'Energy zigzagged across the room'

The local farmer spent the first part of January busily repairing buildings, fences and machinery and I embarked on the essential maintenance work needed to get my body in the best possible shape for the planting that lay ahead. It was time for the first of my fertility prescriptions – a yogic detox.

I arrived to find Kiki one heck of a frustrated yogi, unable to get into The Lotus Room car park – where parking was strictly for teachers only. She was shouting after the woman who'd evidently taken the last place and was now well on her way to the sanctity of John Lewis.

'If you don't get back here right now,' screamed Kiki, 'I'll let your tyres down, bitch!'

Clearly I wasn't the only one in need of a detox.

Dina introduced herself to ten eager students – eight women and two men – and it was immediately clear that help for the toxic was at hand. With her striking looks, muscular physique and tattoos, she reminded me of the Jivamukti tribe I'd encountered in New York's Union Square. I soon found myself entering detox heaven; each posture flowed seamlessly into the next, the shift in gears from a strong, dynamic form to the soft stillness of the restorative poses accompanied by an exotic soundtrack – perhaps a legacy from Dina's previous life as a music journalist. It's a rare thing for me but I was immediately, as they say in yoga circles, 'in the room' – 'cultivating breath and body awareness', releasing my hips and lower back, synchronising my breath with movement, ending the class feeling calm and relaxed, yet deeply energised.

Two and a half hours after we began a thoroughly cleansed Kiki and I floated out of The Lotus Room and wafted our way down the street to The T Lounge, a local café. We spent a happy hour devouring soup and peppermint tea with some of the other students. Sitting at a big long wooden table the conversation opened up into stories about alleged partner-swapping amongst some London-based yoga teachers who were followers of Paul Lowe, an Osho devotee who believed in using sex as a route to enlightenment. What was the selection procedure? Did they pick bike-lock keys out of a Tibetan bowl?

We wondered if our yoga classes, supposedly a safe space in which to peel back layers of ego, were being used as a springboard into peeling back layers of clothing. What was going on? Did the teachers check out your body-fat levels? Check out the tightness of your *Mula Bandha*? I told the story of the glamorous sixty-something divorcee who measured the success of her facelift by the invitation she soon afterwards received to go to one such party. At least these sharing folks had good taste; David had also been asked to come to 'sharing' evenings, though thankfully he hadn't been tempted. I was very relieved when he told me he thought it was all the 'same old, same old – that typical male fantasy of guys wanting to get their rocks off with whomever in the full knowledge of their wife or girlfriend (so they can say they are being honest) while not liking it if their partners do the same.'

One of the male students at the table thought 'it would be great in the short term but in the long run I would be risking the steadfast love of the person who I want to grow old with, who is the mother of our child, my soulmate. My spiritual journey is about trust, truth and doing my duty as a husband and father to the best of my ability... I think you can acknowledge these feelings without acting upon them.'

'I've heard that one of their yoga students has been making a film about a Californian workshop they did together,' I told the assembled crowd. 'Apparently one of the teachers is filmed chatting naked to the camera whilst his also naked girlfriend pleasures him.'

The same male student paused a moment, thoughtfully sipping his green tea. 'Well if they film another one maybe I can be an extra in the orgy scenes,' he mused. 'I don't think that could do anyone any harm.'

Despite the lunchtime conversation, or perhaps because of it, I arrived home feeling serene, gorgeous, and very much myself. I got out of the car, went to fetch my yoga mat and several John Lewis purchases from the boot, and slammed the overhead door on my head. I slammed it so hard that I fell to the ground. I knew I was still alive because I howled like a dog, for about an hour. Then, still with David clutching a bag of frozen peas to my head, we had a row over my decidedly ungreen decision to put three popadoms in our range oven. So much for the detox. Perhaps the practice had moved some blocked energy – apparently this sometimes manifests negatively before healing can begin. As Dina counselled, 'Yin yoga can take you to some quite deep places so it's worth being gentle with yourself afterwards.' What toxins had escaped from my hips or joints that would've made me slam a car door on my head? Whatever it was it was evil. Perhaps I should ring the Dom – get him to come over and exorcise me. Clearly there was a lot of work to do if my body was to become a pure vessel ready to receive a child.

I was a big fan of acupuncture – it seemed the most robust, the most clinically proven of alternative treatments and I'd already had first-hand experience of its ability to heal. Just one session at a centre on the Finchley Road had restored me from the weak wreck that had presented herself there with a cough and cold of three months' duration (ironic given that I was, at this point, Saving the World from Germs) to ninety-five per cent capacity. Five sessions later and I'd never felt better. Two years on and I remained, by and large, untouched by the spluttering of others.

I'd heard good things about acupuncture and fertility. Gabriele and Kiki both knew of people who'd had problems getting pregnant but were now proud parents, thanks, they thought, to acupuncture. Kiki's man seemed a good choice because he had a special interest in pregnancy. She'd nicknamed him The Mad Professor, partly because he liked to talk about himself as a 'science man', partly because his electro acupuncture practice utilised a lot of electrodes and wires that he never seemed to be entirely in charge of, and partly because, in big old cardigans and bare feet, he looked like one. He was also, in the best traditions of mad professors, a little shy, his hands remained tucked into his armpits until he needed to use them, and he had a nervous habit of sucking air between his teeth.

He recommended a course of eight treatments and we soon settled into a comfortable routine. I'd ring the bell of his Edwardian villa every Thursday morning and, without further ado, lie down on the treatment table in front of a roaring fire. The first time he inserted needles into my knees, ankles, elbows and right ear he'd explained that acupuncture would help me to relax, stimulate my hormones and get the energy flowing freely. My body's biochemicals would be mobilised, electrical balances would be restored. He'd clipped wires to each of the needles – apparently running an electric current through them would speed up the process, increasing their effectiveness. I wondered if I might have a Dr Frankenstein moment in which crackling electrical machines combined with thunder and lightning would send me rocketing out into the night, having strangled the unfortunate professor. As it was the machinery suffered a momentary technical hitch, and I felt nothing – either that or I was numb to all feeling. Several minutes of plugging and unplugging wires followed and eventually I felt a gentle electrical pulse coursing through my limbs.

That week and all the weeks following, it was always the same – the Mad Professor plugged and unplugged and replugged, then, when he'd finally succeeded in calibrating the current, he sat down opposite me and we chatted for half an hour. I picked his brains on the local area because he'd been here for most of his life. He introduced me to the work of long-time Beccles resident Adrian Bell (father of war correspondent Martin Bell), whose trilogy of books about farming in the 1930s were instant best-sellers, and for whom the council had erected a blue plaque in Northgate. He introduced me to the delights of walking along the banks of the River Deben with a story about a just-hatched duckling. He'd brought it home because it had no parents or siblings, and Deben the duck lived in the garden for sixteen years, in happy coexistence with a cat, a rabbit, and even, for a short while, a pigeon. He introduced me to the Bear and Bell pub, once owned by a star of *Phantom of the Opera*, *Oklahoma* and *Miss Saigon*, amongst others, and his fella, a council 'waste management executive'. Sadly they'd sold the pub a few months before I stepped across the threshold for a sum that could only be hinted at with an upward rolling of the professor's eyes, and transferred their talents to a country house hotel an hour's drive from Beccles.

I suppose that a bit of me had been hoping for the immediate result that I'd got on the Finchley Road – that I'd leap off the treatment couch after the first session and, not to suggest any moral wrongdoing on the part of the Mad Professor, instantly be with child. Unfortunately I was instantly with period – it arrived two weeks early. 'Was this a good thing?' I asked him anxiously. 'Well we must have stirred things up a bit,' he offered, 'let's wait and see what happens.'

Kate had suggested that I see Melissa – an Ayurvedic practitioner who had just started teaching Kundalini yoga at The Lotus Room. She'd read that Kundalini yoga might be good for fertility and that Ayurveda might also help – 'They believe that women are a pot and you have to keep all the *ojas* – the spiritual energy – standing upright inside.' I didn't know about being a pot but I did know that my time with Dr Kumar in the Ayurvedic wing of Mysore's hospital had helped me get through a very nasty bug I contracted from some water I'd drunk. Ayurvedic medicine is based on the principle of *dharma* – living in harmony with the greater universe and healing based on natural laws; this meant no antibiotics, only pomegranate juice, tablets that tasted suspiciously like coal and Dr Kumar's personal copy of *Harry Potter and the Prisoner of Azkaban*. I decided to go along to one of Melissa's Kundalini classes and check her out – if I liked her I'd ask for an Ayurvedic consultation.

Kate and Kiki met me at The Lotus Room and, together with two other women, we took our first Kundalini class. Melissa sat on her sheepskin rug, a vision in white, her glossy hair a mass of curls, her bright eyes intensely blue in the rays of Monday morning sunshine that cut across her mat. She exuded a robust vitality that made her something of a poster girl for the benefits of Kundalini and Ayurveda, seeming so grounded she appeared to have taken root on her mat. The girl was like an oak tree, one you could curl up underneath and fall asleep, knowing that you'd be safe.

We didn't really know what to expect of the class – none of us Bad Ladies had ever done any Kundalini before and personally speaking I'd always thought of it as wimp's yoga – a few breathing exercises and some meditation. I was in for a shock.

Melissa explained in a strong voice that seemed to issue from some unshakeable and timeless place deep within, that Kundalini yoga is the 'most complete yoga' – 'a yoga of awareness' utilising breath, postures, chanting and meditation.

We got off to a gentle enough start, 'tuning in'.

'Inhale, exhale, inhale, exhale, inhale to begin,'

instructed Melissa, chanting something called the '*Adi* Mantra' to open the class.

'*Ong Namo Guru Dev Namo*,' she sang, in a strong and purposeful voice.

'*Ong Namo Guru Dev Namo*,' we followed.

'This mantra tunes us into the frequency of our higher self or inner master – opening the spiritual channel. Chanting this mantra means that you'll be guided in the practice and you'll be connected to the golden chain of energy that links all the Kundalini teachers and students who have come before us. "*Ong*" is the active aspect of the universe, "*Namo*" is to bow, "*Guru Dev*" is the divine wisdom that draws us from darkness to light – so in this mantra we bow to the divine wisdom of the universe.'

After some 'easy rolls' designed to wake up our spines, Melissa explained that she would be leading us through a precisely timed *kriya* – or series of postures. There would be a different one each week but this first one was designed to strengthen our lungs and balance our lymphatic systems, protecting us against the ill-effects of the January cold snap.

We started off leaning back on our hands and stretching out our legs at a forty-five degree angle to our bodies, bringing our knees into the chest and back out again on the breath. This was hard enough but the addition of *Kapalabhati* or 'bellows breath' made it pretty much impossible, except that Melissa was doing it effortlessly. There was something in her manner that made me understand that failure was not an option so I struggled on.

There followed some madness – the kind of practices envisioned by people who think of yoga as the barmy pursuit of the mentally deranged. The sight of us slapping the palms of our hands on the floor seven times, chanting '*Hut*' each time we slapped, taking care to touch our tongues to the roofs of our mouths on the 't', and sweeping our arms overhead as we yelled '*Hari*!' would have confirmed their worst fears. I only carried on because I knew the door to The Lotus Room was locked and none of these people could get in and, more to the point, I couldn't get out. Also there was the fact that everyone else was doing it, some of them, like Kate, gracefully – what a teacher's pet she was – her hair tracing silvery brush strokes as she tossed her head back on the '*Hari*'. (I was secretly glad when she later confessed that it took her two days to recover from Melissa's classes.)

Our teacher was with us throughout; she reminded me of a particularly purposeful head girl, determined that her girls would do their best. Our persistence had a lot to do with her exhortations. She'd explain what each pose was achieving – in the case of '*Hari*!' it stimulated digestion and more than eighty meridians – and just as you thought you might faint she'd issue words of encouragement:

'Keep going!'

'Nearly there, not too much longer.'

'Any tension just work it out, let it go.'

'You're all doing really well.'

'Use the breath!'

'Last few seconds.'

'Let the emotions come out – happiness, anger, irritation, it doesn't matter – whatever it is. Let it out!'

Each pose would start easily enough, then I'd get halfway through – about five minutes in – and my face would be contorting itself into ugliness good enough to win any gurning competition. There were often tears – partly through sheer physical pain and partly because the *kriya* seemed to be working deep within to release long-held tensions and emotions. Then I'd crash through the pain barrier into the arms of complete euphoria.

The class closed by sealing in this bliss, with a rousing rendition of 'The Sunshine Song', a Gaelic prayer that raised our hearts to the heavens as we wished for the sun to shine on us, love to surround us and pure light to guide us.

The combination of pain and euphoria was really addictive, and that was the clincher. Yogi Bhajan, the man who brought Kundalini yoga to the West, had used this fact to his advantage. He'd seen the hippies of sixties California searching for answers, altering their state of consciousness through drugs, and wanted them to know that they could achieve this ecstasy naturally, through Kundalini – which, according to the website kundaliniyoga.org.uk, means 'the curl of the lock of hair of the beloved' – a somewhat opaque metaphor for 'the flow of energy and consciousness that already exists within each one of us'. He took the decision to go public on what had been an oral tradition for more than fifteen centuries, giving his first lecture in a Los Angeles high-school gym on 5 January 1969. Not a single person came but, undeterred, he declared that 'happiness is your birthright' to an empty hall, and the 'Happy, Healthy, Holy Organisation', '3HO' for short, was born. Shortly thereafter busloads of hippies arrived (did they ever travel any other way?) and the movement got underway. It was easy to see why he was such a hit in sixties' California. The bearded and turbaned six-foot-three Sikh was one cool dude, he was a champion of annual women's camps that turned 'chicks into eagles' and he retained a keen interest in business, acting as a management consultant to his students. Under his tutelage they created Yogi Teas, now a multi-million-pound business and one of the world's leading tea companies, Sun and Son computer systems and Akal security – now the largest judicial security contractor in the USA.

We walked through the centre of Norwich to Melissa's treatment rooms (I'd decided about five minutes into the class that I wanted an Ayurvedic consultation) and as we talked it became clear that Melissa, BSc, PGDip, MSc, was a yogic overachiever. She hadn't loved her course in management with Russian as much as she'd hoped and so she decided to fulfil her childhood dream and practise medicine, doing her masters in Ayurveda at the University of Middlesex and in India. 'Fortunately I love studying,' she enthused, 'and I love researching. I'm never happier than when I'm learning something new – when I was studying Ayurveda I also had a full-time job so I was working seven days a week.' She was now in the final stage of training to become a Kundalini teacher. 'In fact I've just got back from a "White Tantra" workshop – it was amazing – energy zigzagged across the room connecting us to each other, and to Yogi Bhajan,' she explained. No mean feat as Yogi Bhajan had been dead more than ten years. She may have joked that her younger brothers called her the Angel Wah Wah 'after all the silly-sounding mantras' she did, but, by the time we arrived at her treatment rooms, it was clear that Melissa was one of Yogi Bhajan's fully fledged eagles. I determined that if I could exhibit one tenth of her strength and vitality I would surely awaken my inner fertility goddess.

We sat down in the treatment room and the Angel Wah Wah immediately got out her notebook, steadily working her way through more questions about my health than I'd ever been asked before. She found patterns in things I'd never connected – apparently my poor eyesight was related to my low energy levels and a furry tongue. She concluded, half an hour later, that my '*Rasa*', the juice that the digestive system extracts to create vital energies, and bodily functions like pregnancy, was low. 'We need to cleanse your body of its old residual armour – its toxicity – improve the digestive and metabolic processes so that you can absorb the nutrients from food properly.'

There followed a long discussion about my diet. I think she was secretly horrified but she remained very polite. Out went the bar of Galaxy a day, out went my breakfast of yogurt ('too cooling') and bananas ('too sticky'), and out went alcohol altogether. In came a breakfast of porridge with cinnamon, raw cane sugar or stem ginger. I was to have my main meal at lunchtime and make it a big meal – chicken, fish, duck or even pheasant – I'd told her about the Sheriff's gifts. She encouraged me towards warm food and nourishing spices, towards daal and basmati rice, which should be cooked in ghee (to break down unwanted low-density lipids). My evening meal should be lighter – some soup would be ideal – and she prescribed a hefty dose of crumble to replace those cravings for chocolate – she especially recommended apple or pear crumble, and, for a bit of variety, I could try baked apple with raisins. This was the best prescription I think I've ever received – imagine if the NHS prescribed apple crumble – there'd be no problems with patient compliance then.

'By the way,' I asked as I got up to leave, keen to fill in my projected timeline towards conception, 'how long will it take to work if I do the herbs and follow the diet?'

'At least two months.'

'That long?' I whined, dismayed.

'You would find it very difficult to get pregnant in your current state,' said the Angel Wah Wah sadly. 'The only way to speed up the process would be *Pancakarma*.'

'And what would that consist of?' I asked.

'I'd come to your house every day, prepare your meals for you and for the first four days you'd have a full body massage and steam therapy. On days two, three and four I'd also give you *Takara Dhara*.'

I'd had this treatment in India – it was the closest thing to heaven on earth – in which a medicated decoction is poured across the forehead continuously for what feels like an eternity.

'Day five would be a rest day and day six would be Purgation Day – you'd take a herbal drug and expect to pass between eight and ten motions. You should feel light and strong at the end of it,' said the Angel Wah Wah confidently.

I hoped that I would, though based on my only other experience of passing eight to ten motions – in that Mysore hospital – other feelings seemed more likely.

Days seven and eight would be special diet days which would rekindle my digestion, and then the worst bit – I'd have five days of enemas 'to improve the quality of the uterus'.

The Angel finished the consultation by sliding a piece of paper across the table. On it were detailed a number of rules:

- No alcohol
- No strenuous movement or exercise, not even yoga
- No exposure to any form of stress, no violent TV
- No exposure to cold winds
- No travelling in vehicles
- No sex
- No sleeping during the daytime
- No suppression of natural urges (i.e. sneezing, urinating etc)

I decided to take the Angel's apple crumble prescription instead – knowing that I was settling for the slow train to fertility.

12

'The half always catches the hare'

February was a quiet month devoted almost entirely to my fertility quest and, when I wasn't on the Mad Professor's couch or on my yoga mat shouting '*Hut Hari*', I was in the kitchen. I was lucky to have the best ingredients close to home. Des our plumber, owner of Pubic the Terrier and several chickens, gave us the best eggs I'd ever had – their yolks were a thick golden yellow and they tasted so rich, so intensely eggy, that I lost all interest in the supermarket's pale imitations. My herbs – rosemary, mint, sage and chives – came from the decommissioned horse trough outside the kitchen window. My meat came from the next field courtesy of the Sheriff, or from Seppings, where the award-winning sausages were handed over by hardy men whose cheeks were as red as their mince. I bought my vegetables and organic apple juice from a bunch of young women swaddled against the cold in Fresh and Fruity and most of all I looked forward to Beccles' farmers' market – to Goulborn's pies, piping hot cups of tea and the smell of bacon and onions sizzling on the giant fryer.

Food became my medicine – the soothing relaxation

that comes with creaming butter and sugar, watching rasp-berries melt into porridge, the nurturing smell of grated oranges, lemons and limes, of fried pancetta in a pheasant stew. I'd lost my taste for ready meals, for doing anything quickly; my favourite dish was risotto – coating every grain of rice with liquid, waiting till each ladle was absorbed, inhaling the rich aroma of porcini, home-grown sage and garlic; an exercise in slow.

I continued to see Kiki and Kate at their classes and they often joined me for Kundalini on a Monday morning, Kate cementing her position as the teacher's pet and Kiki and me struggling at the back. The classes were, more often than not, followed by a catch-up in nearby Café 33, fighting to make ourselves heard over the hiss and scrape of the coffee machine. There, over mugs of green tea and porridge, we'd get our diaries out and make plans – a *Sex and the City* night on Kiki's capacious sofa, a trip to see Goldfrapp or the Buena Vista Social Club organised by Kate, who was always first off the block booking tickets, thanks to her subscription to every online ticket alert in the county.

One foggy Friday night we met at the Assembly Rooms in the centre of Norwich – a grade I Georgian building in which the Norfolk gentry used to party and network. We were there, at Kate's instigation, to see the promisingly titled Bliss – a duo specialising in 'healing', 'spiritual' music. This evening, in place of the landed gentry, the chandelier-laden, peach-panelled room was filled with a different kind of elite – Norfolk's rainbow-clad movers and shakers. The Bad Ladies, despite adherence to a different dress code, knew quite a few of the assembled New Age gentry and set about introducing me to tarot readers, massage therapists and Shamanic healers. Through them I gathered that there was much anticipation of Lucinda's 'blissed-out' voice which apparently enabled a person to 'travel beyond emotions to a space that is tonal, that is unchanging' and of the pianist, who'd risen from the Sheffield steel works to a residency with Simply Red. The rainbow-clad and those of us who preferred our colours to occupy separate garments sat together in a long row, there were lots of jokes about how hand *mudras* enable one to hold several glasses of Pinot Grigio at the same time, but I sat sipping my sparkling water and quietly polishing my halo, which seemed fitting given song titles like 'A Hundred Thousand Angels' and 'Come into the Light'.

I thought I'd never heard their music before but Kate assured me that she often played their soft dreamy songs; and as soon as Lucinda Drayton, a blonde wannabe mermaid in a ribbony emerald-green silk top and trousers, started singing I recognised them and, by the end, though I struggled a bit with talk of angels 'appearing at traffic lights', I was fairly sure I'd had a brush with the 'space that is tonal, that is unchanging'.

Afterwards the blissed-out Bad Ladies repaired to Baba Ghanoush for brown rice salad and a catch-up. We started with a status update from Kate. I was well on the way to discovering that she was built in the same way as a swan – the chilled-out surface masked the hard work that was going on beneath. Besides the eight yoga classes she taught every week and the monthly workshops at The Lotus Room, she had started giving twice-weekly privates to Lady Birkie, who was proving surprisingly adept for a woman in her fifties (something to do with having an It Girl mother and being whisked off to India in the sixties to follow in the footsteps of the Beatles), and had taken on an extra class teaching restorative yoga to the recovering drug addicts of Great Yarmouth. Unsurprisingly she was knackered.

'I just don't think I've got the work–life balance sorted out,' she said. 'I was cleaning out the car the other day and I realised, as I fished out sandwich wrappers, paper cups and even a blanket, that I spend half my life in it, charging up and down the A146 to and from classes and the office. It's not the way we meant it to be, there's no time for anything and I'm not even seeing Will because three nights out of five I'm teaching yoga until nine. He does all the cooking and clean-ing the house and walking the dogs and I don't think that's fair when he's also got work to do.'

'Is there anything you can give up?' I asked, concerned. I didn't want my friend burning out as I had back in my mid-thirties.

'Not the way things are set up at the moment, no. I think we're just going to have to speed up the Ibiza plan; go out there in March, talk to the committee who run the place, see what we can work out.'

'Well, take it slowly,' I counselled, 'don't rush into anything.'

I was worried for her, was this really the right thing to do? It seemed like such a big step – they were a Spanish-speaking community and although most of them spoke English too it was still another country. There was something about Kate which was, despite the Ibiza Girl dress code, very English.

'So, Lucy,' said Kate, changing the subject, 'what's the latest on the fertility quest?'

'It's going *really* well, thanks to all your advice – no result to report yet but I've been off the Pinot Grigio for six weeks now and I feel a lot better, I've even been singing the Angel Wah Wah's "Sunshine Song" around the house.'

'And how's David dealing with it?' asked Kiki.

'Well, I think David still prefers country and western music but he's happy to let me get on with the plan and is very supportive – he's even given up drinking too. He seems more relaxed – he's really enjoying being up at the house – he comes up every Thursday night now because he loves it so much and I love watching him, my King of the Kitchen, crowned with his tweed cap, sitting at the head of the table dispensing business advice and cups of tea to the locals.'

'Wasn't he giving your plumber some help when I came over the other day?' asked Kate.

'Yes, and his most recent recruit is a tattooed and muscular tree surgeon whose similarly lithe cousin just happens to be Godfrey Devereux.'

'Not the pony-tailed yoga guru whose preference for practising in a tiny loin cloth is legendary in yoga circles?' asked Kiki.

'The very same,' I said gleefully.

'Does he have the same body?' asked Kiki, coming over all unnecessary.

'Not sure,' I replied, 'he looks pretty toned in his jeans and T-shirt but thankfully he didn't trim our willow tree in his knick-knacks.'

'Can you introduce me?' asked Kiki, spurting out the words.

'Slow down, Bad Lady,' I said, laughing, 'I'm afraid that he's married.'

Despite this blow Kiki remained on fine form; she'd done her detox, decided that the soulful cruiser didn't have enough going on between his ears for a long-term relationship, chucked him and celebrated by spending Valentine's Day on a date with a film producer she'd met on *Guardian* Soulmates.

'He's clever, handsome and talented and, unlike Prawn Man, he's actually interested in *me*,' she said triumphantly. 'We ended up talking about my film ideas – he was really interested in one about a forties swing band.'

'Sorry, back up, Bad Lady – your film ideas?' I asked, fascinated. 'I knew you liked watching films but I didn't know you wrote them...'

'Oh yes,' said Kiki, '*The Devil Wears Prana, Mat Wars: Episode Six, A New Drishti* and *Gokulam Hills 90210* chronicling a bunch of Western yogis' adventures in Mysore's most fashionable post code – they're all mine. But seriously, my masters was in Film Studies and prior to becoming a yoga goddess I was in fact a lowly and humble scribe for a film magazine – it was a galley ship of slaves but I stuck it out and worked there as a sub-editor for years. Around that time I developed some screenplay ideas – I just never quite managed to get any of them off the ground. I think I just needed someone to encourage me, to invest in me. Who knows, perhaps he is The One.'

'Is there no end to your talents?' I asked, marvelling that someone could not only look brilliant in a pair of hyper pink leggings at the age of forty-three, be a great yoga teacher, have an MA, a PhD in progress, several film scripts in the works, and three children – all in the same time it had taken me to grow up, find a man and move to Norfolk.

'I guess I've let my inner film buff get a bit muffled by my yoga goddess but I really feel excited by this idea and it all feels very serendipitous and cosmic and like the purpose of it all, really.'

And with this Kiki jumped up and gave us a demonstration of giros, barridas and ochos that had us all, and our fellow diners, mesmerised.

The next day, on a freezing cold but bright Saturday, I forwent the comforts of our kitchen to observe riders and horses setting off on a hunt. This was at the invitation of the Sheriff who saw it as a valuable part of my training for life in the country. We met in the backyard of a nearby farm where the Sheriff's wife was handing out beakers of port and hot sausages cooked in honey and ginger. It took a great deal of effort on both our parts to say no to the port but we managed it – the same could not be said for the sausages.

The first thing I noticed, after the port and sausages, was the strict colour coding – the Sheriff was back in his yellow teddy bear tie and matching yellow socks, the Masters of the Hunt, including the Squire, wore green jackets, the other riders wore black or tweed. Everyone was impeccably turned out – the white jodhpurs were Persil white, the black boots shone in the sunlight. I mentally awarded my best-dressed prize to the older gentleman who arrived on horseback in a long black jacket and bowler hat.

Just as I'd enjoyed the tribal nature of the pheasant shoot, I enjoyed the camaraderie of the hunt, even found myself wanting to belong here, to be rocking the green jackets and white jodhpurs look, but instead I was in jeans, a pea coat and a rather fetching Fair Isle knit beret. David may have worn an old leather jacket and jeans but at least his tweed cap was right. Once again my tribal aspirations came unstuck with the subject matter; I didn't have any inclination to ride, much less to own a horse, and I was still thinking of turning our stables into a yoga studio. On top of my lack of equine chemistry there was the issue of killing the 'quarry' – although it had been banned in the Hunting Act of 2005 the hunt still had all those associations, and saboteurs had been known to attempt the removal of the Sheriff's jacket in protest. I settled into the easy role of spectator knowing that my spiritual homeland lay firmly with yoga and The Bad Ladies.

The horses were as impeccably dressed as their owners. Christine, the stylish driver of the beaters' wagon I'd met back in November, was the first to arrive on her horse, a pretty grey. Her horse sported an immaculate mane which, she told me, had taken her all of the previous evening to plait. I thought this activity might've given her an extra hour in bed but apparently she still had to get up at 6.30 to make all the final preparations. She was much occupied by the correct adjustment of her stirrups. 'Are they level?' she asked us, standing up in the saddle in the manner of Arabella Weir doing 'does my bum look big in this?' Another woman rode a horse with a red ribbon in its tail – I was just about to go over and pat its hind legs – until I learned that the red ribbon denoted that the horse was a kicker. Clearly he was a bit of a handful – I watched his rider struggling to gain control, eventually deciding that she needed both hands on the reins and therefore needed to take the plastic beaker of port between her teeth in the manner of a horse's bit.

The Sheriff introduced us to the 'Huntsman', the man in charge of the dogs – sorry, I mean 'hounds'. He looked like a champion jockey to me – a small man with a handsome weathered face and something of the Italian about him, dark brown eyes and an olive skin. We learned that it was a job he'd been born into. His father and grandfather had been Huntsmen before him, and today his son, his apprentice, stood by his side, listening politely as I ploughed my way through the key questions as they occurred to me.

'How many hounds will be taking part today?' I asked.

'Nine pairs and a half,' he explained.

'A half?'

'Yes, the half always catches the hare,' he told me.

I nodded in the manner of one who had understood.

'It's a tradition,' he said, clarifying.

'And what kind of hounds will you be using today?' I asked, moving on.

'Today we are using harriers because they stand twenty-one shoulder high.'

I raised my eyebrows quizzically.

'We match the height of the hound to the quarry so we have different hounds for different quarry. The harrier at twenty-one shoulder is a medium-sized dog so it's ideal for hunting hares. We use bigger dogs for foxes.'

I was feeling a bit confused. Since killing had been banned why bother with different heights of dogs? They were only following a dead hare's scent.

'We're maintaining the tradition until the Conservatives get in and repeal the law,' explained the Sheriff. 'Which of course it will be – it's the most humane way of controlling the population of hares, foxes and mink – only the lead hounds execute the quarry, and death is almost instantaneous.'

We watched the riders walk round to the front of the

farm until thirty or more horses stood in a circle overlooking the valley. It was a timeless scene – riders and horses standing high above the flat marshes and meadows – we might have been back in 1534 when the first fox hunt took place. David and I watched them cantering off – admiring the red lining of the hunting jackets flapping in the wind. We looked at each other and shivered – David's eyes were watering against the biting cold wind. It was a shame we couldn't partake of the central heating known as port – as we walked back to the car I noted that those thirty riders, and their helpers, had got through fourteen bottles in less than an hour – well, it was a *very* cold day.

13

'Power up your earth chakra'

The first time I witnessed duck rape was on Beccles quay. There I was enjoying a beautiful March morning, the sky a deep blue, the boats bobbing gently on the water, everything peaceful in my world, when suddenly rounding the corner I came across a huge white drake with what looked like red mould over its face – ugly did not begin to describe it – and its beak was firmly wrapped around a poor duck's neck.

'Well, she isn't going anywhere fast,' said the old lady sitting on the bench.

'It looks quite rough,' I said, 'do you think she's all right? Should we step in?'

'Best let nature take its course,' she said. 'Ducks are always getting raped by the drakes – that's just the way they are – but don't worry dear, she gets her own back, she'll just eject his business if the experience wasn't to her satisfaction.'

I came home to find a duck hobbling around our garden, presumably she'd also been the victim of domestic violence. 'Yep, the old boys can be quite rough,' said Bill our gardener, 'sometimes a bunch of 'em will even gang rape and some of the old gerls get drowned as a result.'

Their early couplings might have been violent but once the drake had achieved his objective he was love's young dream personified. I'd stand at the kitchen window and watch him following her attentively across the lawn; there was symmetry in their movements – sitting equal distances from the pond, moving up and down the garden path in perfect harmony – I wondered idly if I could popularise Synchronised Ducks as a new sport.

The ducks weren't the only ones bringing forth new life – the fields were full of lambs and calves, the hedges and meadows, a dirty shade of brown for the past six months, turned yellow, purple and white overnight. Bluebells and dandelions carpeted the woodland floor. Daffodils were ubiquitous – forming circles of yellow round the base of willow trees, for sale on roadside tables, and even finding a place on the social calendar – I picked up leaflets for Daffodil Days at neighbouring halls and schools and detected a certain amount of daffodil snobbery – as Lady Birkie put it, 'Why go and look at other people's daffodils when one has plenty of one's own?'

Once again, as nature's cycle continued, I couldn't help but wonder why everything else was capable of reproducing, everything except me. I worked hard to remain open to the possibility that it would happen, and continued to put my energy into The Bad Ladies, cooking and yoga.

The Angel Wah Wah was on top form, her classes bursting with spring themes. We'd finished boosting our immune systems in February and now we moved on to dispelling fear, and opening to opportunities. The 'Green Energy Set' 'is a *kriya* to open our hearts and attract the prosperity we deserve', explained the Angel Wah Wah. I wondered if it was a green energy set because green is the colour of money but wisely she reminded us that 'prosperity can come in different forms' and explained that 'green is the colour of the heart *chakra* and the colour of creativity'.

As we lifted our bottoms, and dropped them onto the floor, I thought about creating a prosperous second *chakra*, abundant with fertility, but it has to be said that all our drops became more convincing when our Angel told us that it was 'great for cellulite'. We squatted on the ground and extended our hands straight out in front of us, our fingers interlaced and forefingers 'pointing out to infinity' as we breathed like fire bellows. The Angel Wah Wah explained that this was a great one for anger management. 'My boss at the time made me furious, so I squatted down behind my desk and did this pose for ten minutes and I was restored to perfect calm.'

It was a powerful class; we bowed to the Infinite, we made Cosmic Connections with our hands in Venus Lock above our heads, we produced green energy by chanting '*Hari Hari Hari Hari*' for ten minutes. Afterwards we retired to Café 33 for a restorative bowl of porridge. Perhaps it was 'The Sunshine Song', perhaps it was the daffodil parties, perhaps it was the boundless blue skies; but we were all pursuing our purposes with renewed energy that March.

Kate was making a lot of effort to slow down, having massages and going on 'chilled out' Simon Low yoga workshops. She rather destroyed the image of a relaxed weekend with tales of speed walking, claiming that Simon walked faster than she, but I wasn't convinced. Kiki was also speed walking through life – her film producer had turned out to be a flake who used techniques not dissimilar to those of the casting couch so she was redirecting her energies into teaching and her PhD, she'd found a new, more advanced Argentine Tango teacher in Norwich and had celebrated by perusing slinky numbers worthy of a Buenos Aires hottie in Top Shop, or 'Tosho' as she liked to call it. She announced that she was also working on a range of Mysore-inspired yoga practice T-shirts – 'Always *Mula Bandha*' in the 'Always Coca-Cola' style being the launch leader. We selflessly volunteered to try out the prototype.

I updated The Bad Ladies on my progress. 'I'm still eating plenty of crumble and still seeing the Mad Professor who's still wearing the same woolly jumper. The fire roars in the grate despite the fact that it's March and he's still having problems with his circuits – last week I told him I'd buy him new plugs if he got me pregnant, so to speak. It's all going well except that,' I paused, 'I can't shake the feeling that I'm just sitting around waiting for something to happen.'

'I can understand that,' said Kate sympathetically, 'my friend Ali, the yoga for fertility expert from London, is coming up to stay with me for the weekend, would you like to see her for a consultation? Her husband is a hypnotherapist and he could see you too if you were interested – could be useful if you want to understand if there's anything in your unconscious mind that's stopping you from getting pregnant.'

The following Saturday morning found me knocking on the door of Kate's house in Harleston. A man who looked much like a teddy bear opened the door. He had lots of hair and big round eyes, his lineless face the shape of a big heart. His square body hung from broad shoulders clothed in a thick bottle-green jumper and he had the curious combination of looking very strong and very soft all at the same time.

'You're not Kate,' I said, stating the obvious.

'Kate has gone out with my wife,' said The Bear, 'they've taken our baby for a walk. Come in and let's get started.'

I followed him as he padded down the corridor to Kate's sitting room. We set ourselves up on the floor, me on a large white bean bag and him on an Indian rug, cross-legged in lotus pose. Skeins of incense curled their way slowly towards a Moroccan light suspended from the ceiling.

I explained my quest.

He considered me, thoughtfully. 'Candle gazing is a very powerful thing,' he said, 'let's do that.'

I felt vaguely disappointed – I'd hoped for something a little more hi-tech – I'd imagined falling into a trance and reliving the moment of my delivery, awakening joyful in rebirth.

He lit a candle in the corner of the room. 'Sit less than an arm's length away from the candle and make yourself comfortable on the bean bag,' he instructed me.

I sat with my back to The Bear, feeling rather like my seven-year-old nephew Teddy, stuck in the Naughty Corner.

'Look into the main body of the flame just above where the wick is,' he instructed. 'Look with your eyes open – have an unwavering gaze, don't blink until your eyes start to water, then close your eyes and look at the after-image of the flame. Do *Ujjayi* breathing.'

I dutifully contracted my throat and began to make the sound of the ocean with my breath.

'Listen to that sound. Your awareness is travelling to the flame on the exhale and on the inhale your awareness is travelling back to your forehead. Do this three or four times. The after-image is much more important than the flame itself.'

He left me for about ten minutes after which I returned to face him.

'How do you feel?' he asked me gently.

I hadn't been conscious of much happening but I suddenly felt very flat. 'I feel sad, and tired,' I admitted, my eyes watering.

'It's natural,' said The Bear comfortingly, 'it's a powerful practice – one of the six cleansing practices in Hatha Yoga. As you practise things will become clearer; you will get a sense of what is rocking the boat. Start with just ten minutes and build up gradually to twenty.'

I agreed that I would.

'Let's do a heart *mudra* now, a womb meditation,' he said encouragingly, 'it will power up your earth *chakra*.'

He instructed me to sit with my first finger curled into the base of my thumb, the second and third fingers connecting with the top of my thumb and my little finger sticking out.

After a few minutes he asked me to shift my left hand on to my heart and my right hand on to my belly. 'Start your *Ujjayi* breathing again. Breath travels up on the inhale and down on the exhale. Imagine that you are shaped like a pot – this will help you direct the flow of energy. Just allow yourself to open up, imagine your Fallopian tubes opening. Tilt your head to the left to listen to your heart.'

Nothing happened to begin with. My thoughts wandered to Ali and what was to follow, to David and what he would think of my morning pursuits, to what we would eat for dinner. Then there was stillness. And suddenly there was my child – an eighteen-month-old laughing boy with a thick mop of black hair, big brown eyes and long eyelashes, held tight in my arms. We were on a safari in India and he was pointing at the elephants and laughing with great glee. He clearly thought the whole thing was hilarious. I clutched him tight to my chest, felt the warmth of his head, and inhaled the smell of him – his hair, his cotton shirt mixed with sweat and dust. Nothing had ever smelled better, it was a smell that took me home to myself, and in that moment I understood what it is to be a mother.

I sat quietly, silent tears pouring down my face.

Afterwards I explained my vision to The Bear. 'Was that a memory?' he asked gently.

'No, I've never been on a safari. What surprised me was that my son had such a strong personality,' I said, smiling, 'he clearly loved the adventure, and the heat.'

'It's amazing how developed baby's personalities are,' agreed The Bear. 'They are born with a very strong sense of self. You know, some mums have a real dialogue with their unborn children.'

I looked at my stomach and was surprised to see that I wasn't already six months pregnant.

The Bear explained the importance of this visualisation. 'There is a lot of evidence to suggest that if we think of something as real at the unconscious level it becomes real. Whatever it is – goal setting, publishing a book, even having a baby – your intuition picks up on things and makes it real – it's an energetic lock that's happening.'

Just at that moment there was a knock at the door and a woman with a damp elfin face and steamed-up glasses entered the room.

'Hi, I'm Ali,' she announced cheerily, rubbing herself dry with a towel. 'It's raining outside, if you hadn't guessed.'

She took off her coat to reveal a soft purple tunic and a small golden OM necklace and we got down to business immediately. My hour-long yogic journey towards fertility started in supported *Savasana* with a bolster beneath my knees, making *Yoni mudra,* my hands in a diamond shape four or five centimetres below my tummy button.

'Breathe deeply into the abdomen,' instructed Ali, kneeling down beside me. '*Yoni mudra* will help you build female energy and open *Svadistana chakra* – the seat of creation.'

Ali removed the bolster and, keeping my hands in the same position, I tilted my pelvis slowly towards me, peeling my spine off the floor. Exhaling on the way up, and inhaling on the way down.

'Beautiful,' said Ali.

She watched over my every move – I began to feel as a pregnant woman might, as if my body was bearing precious cargo and every move must be measured against its worth.

She moved me gently into a supine *Baddha Konasana* – the soles of my feet touching, my knees wide apart. Once again I lifted my hips slowly towards the ceiling.

'You have great mobility,' said Ali, 'that enables us to get beyond the physical body – *Ana Mayakosha* – to work on the second level – on the *Prana Mayakosha* – the energy body.'

I was beginning to feel awesome.

'Let's stir the porridge,' said Ali, smiling.

I sat upright, my legs in front of me, slightly apart.

'Imagine that you are holding a large wooden spoon,' said Ali.

This was going to help me get pregnant?

'There's a big bowl of porridge in between your legs. Your job is to stir the pot.'

'Okay,' I said, laughing.

'Now, keeping your arms at shoulder height, lean forwards from the hips and start to make circular motions, use soft *Ujjayi* breathing to inhale as you lean back, exhale as you move forward over your feet.'

I stirred my porridge until all the oats had been absorbed and I had a good creamy texture.

'Beautiful,' admired Ali. 'You are ready for the *Chandra* sequence – the Moon sequence. It will energise and release your pelvic bowl.'

I thought this might be the point at which I got to my feet, but no, this sequence was performed on the knees. Employing *Ujjayi* breath once again I came to all fours and dipped my spine, looking forwards and up as I inhaled. I tucked my chin into my chest, tucked my tailbone under and sucked my abdomen into my spine as I exhaled.

I swung my tailbone up and into downward dog. I raised my left foot and flexed my foot. I raised my right foot and flexed my foot.

I sank down into Child's Pose – kneeling with my forehead to the floor.

'Beautiful,' concluded Ali.

It was strange, but as someone who hadn't got to her feet in the last hour I felt shattered.

'Let's finish with some *Yoga Nidra*,' said Ali.

Fabulous. *Yoga Nidra* means 'Sleep of the Yogis'. It's not a literal sleep but a deep relaxation.

Ali arranged me in a supported cross-legged position

against the wall – every part of my body in contact with at least one cushion or a bolster.

'I call this the "Pose of the Queen",' explained Ali.

I could see why.

'I am going to leave you for ten minutes. Just relax. Fill your bowl,' she instructed me.

When she returned I was so relaxed I could hardly speak or move. All I could think about was the little boy I had visualised – my playmate on safari. I felt warm and soft, my tummy like a marshmallow. I turned down Kate's invitation to stay for lunch; I wanted to sit with these feelings, and to share them with David. I drove home, past the marshlands and fields of sheep huddling together in the driving rain, feeling like a queen surveying her country, serene in the certain knowledge that a child was possible.

We celebrated Easter with a house full of nieces and nephews – the first sighting of Jessica covered in chocolate and Millie in her candy-pink tights and matching dress had the temperature on my broody-ometer up to four hundred degrees centigrade in the space of a millie-second. On Easter Monday David and I gave the other adults a break and took the children for a walk in the woods. Snow had fallen overnight, carpeting the ground with a four-inch sparkling blue-white crust that delighted the children. We cast the first human footprints amongst the arrow prints of pheasants, the girls wriggled in our arms and Teddy went looking for snowmen, returning to point out that the bracken that stuck up out of the snow looked like the bristles on David's face.

'I'd give anything to have a child right now,' I confessed to David, pulling him closer as Teddy shrieked with surprise

– a hare had shot across the track, leaving deep uneven marks behind it.

'So would I, I'm just worried that I'm going to be too old soon,' said David heavily. 'I'm forty-nine this year and I just don't have the energy I did, I like my sleep too much.'

'So what are you saying?' I asked gently, as much for my sake as for his.

'I'm saying that we should get on with it if we're going to. I don't know, maybe it's my biological clock going off.'

'Men don't have biological clocks,' I retorted impatiently.

'Oh, but they do. I was reading this article the other day and apparently over the age of thirty-five there's a big reduction in our fertility – it's not as much as it is for women but it's there.'

I had no idea. Had tales of Luciano Pavarotti, Warren Beatty and Clint Eastwood achieving fatherhood in their sixties distorted the truth about male fertility, just like all those female celebrities claiming baby joy in their forties?

'But your tests were fine,' I countered.

'I know, but for how much longer? Who knows?'

'So what do you want to do?'

'Let's try IVF,' he replied. 'We're both sick of waiting, why don't we just get on with it?'

'But there's only a four per cent chance of success.'

'It's a chance, Babe.'

'And there's hope in a chance,' I replied, clasping his hand firmly through my thick gloves.

14

'They see the word "sperm" and mistake me for Viagra'

The big question was where to have IVF; could anyone offer me better than four per cent odds? I was pondering this question when I arrived at the Quaker Meeting House the next Wednesday. I took Kate aside after class; did she happen to know of any IVF clinics in Norfolk? She didn't but she knew someone who might and rang me the next day.

'I asked a doctor friend of mine and she said that there isn't one in the whole county. Amazing, isn't it. Apparently the nearest one is Bourne Hall near Cambridge, where someone called Professor Bob Edwards had his practice, she's not sure if he's still there though, he's quite old now.'

Of course, why hadn't I thought of him before? It would be fantastic to be given new life by my old university pal's dad. I rang the clinic the next morning.

'I am sorry,' said Donna, 'Professor Edwards has retired – he's in his eighties now and no longer practising, though he does write for journals and lectures from time to time.'

That was a shame but never mind, I still felt very

comfortable with the idea of using the clinic that he'd been involved with for so long.

Donna and I were halfway through discussing what blood tests I would need for the consultation when she remembered to ask my age.

'I am forty-three,' I said.

'Then I am really sorry, Lucy, but we can't treat you with your own eggs.'

'Why not?' I asked.

'We've had no success with women of your age. '

'But I have an FSH of seven,' I said. My head was beginning to feel like a furred-up kettle again.

'I am sorry, Lucy. We just think it's wrong to take your money when we haven't had any success. Have a think about it and do come back to us if you are interested in egg donation – we can do that up to age fifty.'

'Fifty?'

'Yes, you assume the age of the person whose eggs you are using so it doesn't matter so much how old you are; it's worth thinking about because we have had success rates of thirty-five to forty per cent.'

'I am not interested in egg donation,' I said miserably. 'We want our own child.'

'I understand that. You might find some London clinics that will take you – have a look at the HFEA tables to see who treats older women, and who has the best results.'

I thanked her for her honesty and got on to their website immediately. The Assisted Reproductive and Gynaecology Centre had the highest average rate in the country – at sixty-one per cent their live birth rate was more than double the national average but it had very little experience of treating women of my age – it had performed seven treat-ment cycles with women of forty-three and forty-four and just one had resulted in a live birth. Only the Lister had performed enough cycles to be able to report a reliable percentage – which, unfortunately, remained four per cent. Guys had achieved three births out of twenty-four cycles – the same success rate as the ARGC but at least it had more experience. These were not large numbers but given that I was clutching at straws, it was at least a straw. I rang them and got passed from one person to another, then put on hold for what felt like hours, I had the feeling I was enter-ing a black hole. Eventually I spoke to a nurse – no, they couldn't fit me in for a month. 'I didn't realise we were so busy,' she said, sounding bemused by the packed diary.

A whole month? No. I wanted to get on with things and, to be honest, I was hoping for a more personal approach, so I rang Gabriele and she put me in touch with one of her friends, a woman who'd had a child at forty-seven.

Sarah told me her story over the phone. 'I'd had five rounds of unsuccessful IVF – I even got a "buy one IVF round get one free" deal from a London clinic – and then I went to CERAM in Spain and got pregnant straight away.'

'Using your own eggs?'

'No, I'm telling you this because you need to know the truth but I am not open about it with everyone so please keep it quiet – the clinic told me that at forty-six my eggs were too old so I had egg donation, and I'd just split up with my man so I needed a sperm donor too. They found me both, and the donors were Jewish, like me. The nurse in charge was called Ruth, she'd worked at St Bart's fertility clinic for fifteen years, and because she was English there was no language problem.

The supply of eggs is pretty plentiful in Spain – they understand the importance of family so they are much more prepared to donate than the Brits. Did you know that in the UK you can wait up to three years for an egg?'

I didn't; with a waiting list like that perhaps it was just as well that they took women up to the age of fifty.

'Do you mind me asking you something, Sarah? How do you feel about having had egg donation, now that your son is two?'

'It's weird, sometimes I look at him and feel sad that he's not biologically me but then someone will say to me "he looks just like you" and I have a little giggle to myself, especially as he's gorgeous. Anyway,' she continued, 'I carried him around for nine months, he used my blood to grow and he wouldn't have had life without me so I *am* his mother.'

I could see this – carrying a child was just as important as conceiving it, and the higher success rates were very tempting, but egg donation seemed to raise so many questions: would I tell anyone? Who would I tell? When would I tell? It was a moral maze. I was going to stick to my own eggs if I possibly could.

I rang CERAM the next day and hit it off with Ruth immediately. The woman had a fine sense of humour and we laughed together about being an older chick. 'Don't mention the "A" word,' she joked.

'Have you had much success with older women?' I asked.

Ruth was reassuring: 'We like to take everything on a case-by-case basis so let's just start with some hormone tests and see where you are.'

'But I have an FSH of seven,' I said, my voice tight with frustration.

'I know,' said Ruth kindly, 'it's just that the test was done almost six months ago and things can change. I'll send you an email detailing our prices and some information about our approach, and you can send the hormone results when you have them – I need day two or three FSH, LH, Oestrodial and Prolactin. If you don't get my email be sure to check your Junk mailbox; thanks to the Spam detectors I'm forever ending up in the trash – they see the word "sperm" and mistake me for Viagra.'

My spirits were high, I had a feeling that I'd found my girl – Ruth was knowledgeable, sensible and funny, everything was going to be all right. I started to plan my stay in Marbella – I'd be there for ten days, have the treatment and treat the whole thing like a holiday. All I needed was a good FSH score; I'd been relaxing for months now, eating loads of crumble, putting on weight, having acupuncture, and practising yoga, so it would surely just be a formality – perhaps my FSH levels would even have gone down, maybe to two or three. Awesome.

My doctor got me an appointment with the nurse specialising in fertility at one of the county hospitals. He thought I could get the tests done there and talk through all the options before I made up my mind about Spain. The day of the appointment dawned bright and I sang all the way there, I was looking forward to getting the show on the road. It was a big hospital, as I got lost in the maze of wards that might or might not lead to the fertility clinic I wondered if I'd ever make my way back to my car, let alone get to Spain.

I finally found the clinic, or should I say corridor? I

waited my turn on a narrow vinyl-covered sofa stuffed into a corner and pretended to read my book, too distracted to concentrate. Finally the nurse's door opened and a businesslike woman with stiff red hair called my name.

The nurse sat me down and it became immediately clear that she wanted to apprise me of the gravity of my situation.

'The chances of you conceiving are very, very slim, Lucy, even with IVF.'

'Yes, I know – the chances are four per cent.'

'To put yourself through a very stressful treatment that may not work means you need to have a very good relationship with your partner.'

'My relationship with David is fine and I am sure we can cope with this,' I said confidently, wishing he was there by my side and not stuck in London.

'A lot of my girls fail and you've got to negotiate that – you need to ask yourself, "How will I feel if the treatment doesn't work?"'

'I know I might fail but I want to try,' I insisted, finding all this talk of 'my girls' and 'failure' really irritating, especially as I couldn't be one of 'her girls' because I was too old to be treated on the NHS – by about 100 years.

'Okay, so where are you thinking of having the treatment?' asked the nurse evenly.

'I've had some consultations at the Lister and I really liked Dr Wren but I'd prefer to go to a small place – I really like the people at the CERAM clinic in Spain, they are a bit cheaper than the UK hospitals and they seem to have good success rates.'

'If I were you I would go to the Lister, or consider Birmingham – I know the head of the fertility unit there. Don't go abroad. There's no magical drug that they've got out there that we don't have here.'

'I know that, but I just feel comfortable with CERAM and I think that's important when it can be a stressful process.'

It was clear that I'd made up my mind so we moved on to the blood tests. I gave her the list that Ruth had given me.

She studied the list. 'I can only do these if you're my patient, and you aren't my patient.'

'I wish you'd told me that before,' I said hotly. 'When we spoke on the phone I explained that I would be on day three of my cycle today and I would need the blood tests. I can't wait another month,' I said, my voice rising in panic.

'Okay, Lucy,' said the nurse, taking pity on me. 'I will do your FSH today, but that's the only one you need – it will give a clear indication of your situation.'

'But the CERAM clinic were very specific about what they needed, I won't be able to have the treatment if I don't have the results.'

Eventually, after several more exchanges, the nurse agreed to do the tests.

I left feeling cross; I didn't like all this talk of failure and while I understood that the nurse was trying to protect the precious resources of the NHS I thought paying for a few blood tests was the least they could do considering that we were going to have to foot the bill for IVF and the huge quantities of drugs that I would need as an older woman. I couldn't wait to get away. I drove home thinking about how different it would be in Marbella, I would amble down to the clinic from my simple but chic B&B, share a few jokes with Ruth, have a couple of injections, and then David and I would lie by the pool all day, spend the evenings promenading with the Spanish, getting lost in the narrow streets of the Arab medina, chancing upon a shaded tapas bar.

The following week Kate, Kiki and I went to our regular class with the Angel Wah Wah.

'It's a good time of year to make decisions, to move forward, to get on and do what you need to do and this *kriya* will help you do that because it'll release conscious and unconscious fears.'

My first reaction was that I didn't have any fears – I was going to get great FSH levels and I was going to have a successful IVF treatment.

Releasing our fears turned out to be hard work – the Angel Wah Wah coached us through *asana* that lasted for nine or ten minutes at a time.

We worked on our kidneys and liver with rhythmic rolls of the spine.

'Any tension, just work it out,' coached our Angel. 'Really enjoy the workout the back is getting.'

After a few minutes of this I started to feel quite nauseous, but apparently this was a good thing. 'You might feel sick as the liver releases toxins.'

Eventually, in the last thirty seconds, the burning sensation in the middle of my back gave way to bliss.

We extended our arms up to sixty degrees, our palms facing up, our fingers straight, our thumbs extended. We opened and closed our hands, bringing the fingertips to the palms in rapid movements.

'We'll be here for some time,' coached the Angel Wah Wah. 'This one releases any deposits that we haven't metabolised. It's a wonderful exercise, it takes the toxins back to the kidneys so they can be metabolised and excreted. They can cause arthritis if they're not removed.'

This one quickly became excruciatingly painful but the Angel was by my side.

'If pain is coming it shows you have some deposits.'

I had to stop.

'It doesn't matter if you stop – your intention is there. You get carried by everyone else – that's the benefit of doing it in a group.'

I looked at Kate, she was doing it effortlessly. I started again.

'Keep breathing.'

'Focus on the breath, draw the attention to the breath.'

'You're doing really well. Keep going!'

'Last ten seconds. Save yourself years of agony!'

Seven minutes later I was DOA.

'Well done, well done, well done,' said the Angel Wah Wah.

There was no rest for the fearful; we made fists, curling our thumbs into the mounds of our fingers, punching out as we exhaled.

'Really let go.'

'Fears will leave you on the exhale.'

'You're doing really well.'

We rotated our fists in small circles, we performed crow squats with a straight spine and finally we sat cross-legged, sticking out our tongues.

'Inhale through the mouth, allowing the cool air to waft over your tongue, exhale through the nose. This one works to remove anger and bad moods.'

I sincerely hoped no one was going to walk in on us.

After that we entered a mellow phase, waving our arms to a chant that sounded like 'wah hey guru' on the CD player.

Getting up to leave I was amazed to find I felt great – perhaps it was just relief at the end of an ordeal, but I really did feel fearless. Whatever life had in store for me – bring it on.

Kiki had an errand to run and Kate had a new class to teach so I walked into Norwich city centre alone. There was a chirpy phone message from the nurse that seemed to match the bright sunshine in mood. I settled down on an iron bench opposite the busy market to return her call. This must be good news – she'd said she would send the results to the doctor – obviously the results were so good she wanted to tell me the news herself. I couldn't wait to ring Ruth at CERAM and organise my trip to Marbella. I dialled the number. A small child slept in a pink buggy by my side as her mother slowly ate a sandwich. This could be me soon.

'Hi, it's Lucy Edge here. You have some results for me?' I asked breezily.

'Your FSH is 47.6.'

'What does that mean?'

'You're perimenopausal,' she announced flatly.

Silence.

The mother ate her sandwich.

The baby slept.

'So what does that mean?' I asked, feeling as if I was just about to be sucked out of an airplane.

'Oh, no IVF clinic will take you on with that FSH level,' she replied cheerily.

'Why is that?' I asked. I was out of the plane, spinning out of control, the ground coming up fast.

'Because you won't respond to the drugs,' came the cool reply.

WHACK!

I hit the ground, the plane soared away from me, the noise of the engines ringing in my ears.

The mother ate her sandwich.

The baby slept.

Time passed, I'm not sure how much.

Numbed by the fall to earth I spent the afternoon running errands. I went to choose some floor tiles. Did I want limestone or slate? I stood for half an hour trying to make a decision but no thoughts came to me. I went to John Lewis to look at fabrics for some new curtains. Once again I stared blankly at the reams of fabric, brushing away the attentions of staff with a shake of the head and a turn of the shoulder. I found myself in Marks & Spencer putting juice and an Edamame bean salad in my basket. Then I realised it was no longer necessary to eat soya beans so I went to Prêt A Manger and ordered a large cappuccino with extra caffeine, onto which I poured half a tin of chocolate flakes. I went back to Marks & Spencer and bought a bag of chocolate peanuts and two tubs of chocolate cornflakes.

I returned to The Lotus Room. I needed to get my car but I was blocked in by Kiki and Kate and my phone had run out of battery so I couldn't call them. I sat on the wall preparing to wait what might be the whole afternoon. I closed my eyes and felt nothing, not even the sun on my face.

'Hello, Lucy.'

It was the Angel Wah Wah. Where had she come from? She had the key to The Lotus Room so we let ourselves in and made some peppermint tea as I explained my news. I was surprised how matter of fact I sounded.

'Oh, so perhaps your hormones have regulated themselves,' she suggested.

'Huh?'

'Perhaps the acupuncture is working.'

'Huh?'

'Yes, it's regulated your hormones – it's revealed where you're really at.'

'Oh.'

'I had a similar case once,' continued the Angel Wah Wah, 'a woman who'd stopped menstruating and then, with the help of acupuncture and *Ayurveda*, she started again. It balanced her body too – but with her it went in the other direction.'

'Oh.'

'At least you've looked at your health and are doing all the right things now,' she concluded, looking at me with her most positive face.

I was glad I'd put the bag of chocolate peanuts and two tubs of chocolate cornflakes in the boot of my car.

Kate appeared. She'd been looking for a dress for her sister-in-law's eco wedding. The Angel Wah Wah recommended Primark, I suggested Tosho. Kate was more in favour of Ginger, the local designer shop where she'd found a Max Mara dress but the size eight was too big – could it be taken in? We were wrestling with this issue when Kiki arrived, and we were all free to leave. I could've told Kiki and Kate my news but words failed me, I don't think I could've coped with their kind words, their hugs and kisses. I drove home cramming chocolate peanuts in my mouth.

Later that day I managed to call David and give him the news.

There was a small pause.

'That's cool, Babe,' said David gently. 'How are you feeling?'

'I can't feel anything,' I said, staring out of the window at the rabbits playing amongst the partridges on our lawn.

'At least we know where we are and can get on with the rest of our lives. We aren't defined by whether or not we have children, we have so many blessings – we can max it out, make some money, travel the world, enjoy our freedom – the world is our oyster.'

His words washed over me. I stared out of the window. There was nothing to say.

David spoke into the silence. 'Don't worry about it, Babe. I love you and I'm not going anywhere.'

Moving slowly around the kitchen I made myself a cuppa and sat with the cat, trying to remind myself of all those blessings – David, The Bad Ladies, The Cappuccino Gurus, my nephews and nieces, the beautiful farmhouse – and yet, when I looked down, there were tears on the table.

15

'Jewish Italian eggs – they'd have smarts and style'

My doctor wrote a letter asking to see me. I went a couple of days later, days in which I had done little more than look out of the window in a daze. As always he looked ridiculously healthy – his bright blue eyes shone, his skin gleamed and his muscles flexed hard beneath his blue shirt. On the wall was a photograph of him looking sinewy, proudly sporting a medal for winning a marathon. Next to it was a picture of his pretty wife with their pretty children.

He studied my hormone results. 'This is the reality of women's hormones, I'm afraid, Lucy. After the age of thirty-six your fertility rate goes down – it's like falling off a cliff edge really, by forty-five your biological clock will have more or less stopped. Realistically you stand more chance of a lottery win than getting pregnant at your age. I am sorry but I think it's better to be brutally honest at this point.'

I agreed that it was.

'With an FSH of forty-seven I think it's time for you to think about following other dreams.'

I agreed that it was, and went straight to the Norwich Complementary Therapies Fair to score some more fertility treatments. My reasoning, as far as it went, was simple: miracles happened and I wanted to be one of them.

The fair was held in the Forum, a light-filled horseshoe of steel, zinc and fifteen-metre-high glass. The atrium was filled with 'spiritual counsellors', astrologists and a 'life master' – a cuddly fellow in a pale violet jumper with a shock of silvery grey hair. I perused a Sacred Earth stall selling remarkably well-preserved 'sixteenth-century' shirts, I observed Bluebell giving crystal therapy and stopped to examine Denise's exhibition of 'paintings of magic, love and peace' staffed by a winsome old man with a snow white beard and ponytail – presumably not Denise.

I left armed with the number for a homeopathic endocrinologist, Doreen Virtue's *Archangels and Descendent Masters* 'to establish which Archangels or Descendent Master would help me conceive', and details of a complementary therapy centre on the outskirts of Norwich that I hadn't heard of before.

I spoke to the manager on the phone the next day; Sally told me that they'd had some success in treating infertility.

'One woman had seven miscarriages and now she has a lovely baby,' she said, her voice rich, husky and compelling.

'What treatments did she have?' I asked eagerly.

'I can't remember right now but come in and see me and in the meantime I will think about what will help you.'

So there I was, waiting in one of the sunny therapy rooms taking in my surroundings; a chart detailing the thirty-eight Bach flower remedies, a bookcase stacked with esoteric paperbacks called *Hands of Light, Questions from the*

Heart, The Dancing Wu Li Masters, a bright pink velour dressing gown hanging on the back of the door.

Sally arrived, bringing with her a strong smell of cigarette smoke. She gave me a penetrating look over her glasses, her steely hair in a bun.

'I feel a special connection to anyone suffering from fertility problems as I have been there myself,' she explained, carefully keeping eye contact at all times. 'My first husband had a low sperm count but,' she said, shrugging her shoulders, 'there was no problem with my second husband, and yet, still I didn't fall. A clairvoyant told me he could see three souls who'd come, and gone, that I'd been pregnant three times but that each time I lost it – I knew this myself but he confirmed it for me.'

'I am really sorry,' I said, wondering how these three souls could be divined.

Sally continued, 'Thank you, love. I believe that everything is pre-ordained; that we choose our parents and that this lifetime was given to me to experience freedom. This also was confirmed by the clairvoyant.'

I envied her clarity; she seemed to have considerable self-assurance in an area that seemed to me to be straining at the leash of credibility. 'So why do souls come and go like that?' I asked, trying to understand.

'Because they are here to teach their parents about loss,' she said thoughtfully, 'or because they are old souls who need to finish something off but don't need to be here for long.'

I stared at the pink dressing gown behind her and bit down hard on a tongue which wanted to say 'and sometimes shit happens'.

I needed to change the subject before I blurted out

something inappropriate. 'What would you suggest I do to improve my chances of conceiving?' I asked her.

'I have some ideas for you,' said Sally, laying out what quickly became a bewildering array of leaflets.

'Herbal medicine?'

'Iridology?'

'Aromatherapy?'

'Indian head massage?'

'Emotional Freedom Technique often works where all else has failed,' she explained, 'it's based on the idea that negative thoughts and emotions cause a disruption in the subtle energy body and that these emotions and memories can be released by tapping the appropriate meridians...'

'Metamorphic Technique could be of interest to you, Lucy – the therapist massages your feet, hands and head – releasing any emotional blockages that date from the womb...'

'Or how about Optimum Health Balance Kinesiology?' suggested Sally. 'There's no effort involved – your body tells the therapist what it needs to get pregnant by answering "yes" or "no" to symbolic cards that are placed face down on your tummy.'

'Symbolic cards?'

'Yes. There are symbols for stress, for pain, for vitamin deficiency, there's even one for the ninth dimension.'

'The ninth dimension?'

'The dimension of the universe beyond our personal control – the one that brings into being whatever we wish for,' explained Sally, 'and there's ten per cent off that one this month.'

She handed me a glossy brochure. 'If you want to have several treatments a package would be better value for money.'

I flipped through its pages. Herbal medicine with reflexology and a half-body massage? A full-body massage with Bach flower remedies and crystal healing? I began to feel quite giddy.

'I'm not sure,' I confessed, wearily picking up my coat and bag, 'I need a bit of time to think about it. It's a lot to take in.'

Sally came to the door with me. 'I wish you bliss and love and for everything to turn out as it should.'

I wanted to be open to possibility but please, 'turn out as it "should"'? And whose 'should' was that? When it came to religion I considered myself a liberal, pluralist and tolerant, but still, the idea of a higher authority imposing its will was hard to take.

I got in the car and, as I sunk into my seat, I found that I was totally exhausted, confused and cross. Really cross. All this leaflet gazing seemed to be an elaborate plan to get me to spend money and the treatments all sounded decidedly dodgy to me. I realised that I didn't want to hear about Emotional Freedom or Metamorphic Techniques, I didn't want to read books about Archangels, and I didn't want to eat any more crumble. I was sick of the mystery surrounding New Age therapies and nor did I want anything more to do with Western medicine's cold hard science and statistics; suddenly, for the first time in nine months, I stopped wanting any more fertility treatments. All I wanted was a large glass of Pinot Grigio and my Bad Ladies.

I rang Kiki and we agreed to an emergency summit meeting, scheduled for the following evening. She opened the door of her house dressed in a fuchsia silk salwar kameez and embroidered slippers and I fell into her welcoming arms, burrowing my face in her mane of hair as I sobbed.

'It's all right, Lucy,' she repeated over and over again, rubbing my back.

Kate came to the door and led me into Kiki's kitchen, filling bowls with popadoms and chutneys as Kiki busied herself preparing an Indian feast. It was immediately comforting to be sitting at her table, to see the pink plastic flowers that garlanded the bookcase, the fridge covered with pictures of her children, the film-noir posters on the walls, to feel her cats brushing up against my legs as they competed for attention. We opened a bottle of Pinot Grigio, the windows steamed up with the frying of onions and garlic and we settled into an examination of the events of the past week.

'How are you feeling?' asked Kate quietly.

'I don't know, I think I'm still in shock,' I replied. 'First of all there was the shock of the rocketing FSH score – from seven to forty-seven in six months – how did that happen? Then there was the shock of not being eligible for IVF – I just didn't know these fertility clinics turned people away,' I told them, shaking my head in disbelief. 'I always thought they were greedy and would want to take your money whatever the odds, but I guess, since competition for business is fierce, it's all about the statistics. No one wants an old bird like me dragging their numbers down.'

'It must've felt like having the door slammed in your face,' said Kate, taking care not to dip her embroidered bell-bottom sleeves in the wine as she refilled my glass.

'And I just can't believe that there have been all these scientific advances and none of them will help me,' I said, my voice wobbling. 'It makes me feel like a real failure.'

'You're not a failure, Lucy,' said Kiki firmly, passing me a box of tissues.

'I know that rationally but after I saw the doctor I just went into a tailspin of madness,' I explained. 'I'd always kept my distance from those women who I saw as obsessed about having children. Then, when I found myself talking about a treatment in which my body would read ninth dimension symbolic cards I realised, to my horror, that I was there myself.'

'You're a strong woman, Lucy, you'll come through it, I know you will,' said Kiki, arranging a series of small brass bowls containing the brilliant jewel colours of daal, spinach and tandoori chicken.

'I just don't seem to be able to let go of the dream,' I said, wiping away the snot from my nose.

'It'll take time,' said Kate, handing me another tissue, 'just be patient.'

'There's something else,' I said hesitantly. I hardly dared speak the words. 'David is an accepting man but what impact is all this going to have on our relationship? He might be forty-eight but his sperm is in full working order. He could just walk away, find a younger model – I could lose him – my long-awaited love, my best friend...'

'What has he said about it all?' asked Kate, carefully serving me something from each dish.

'He just tells me he loves me and that he's not going anywhere.'

'So listen to that, Lucy,' said Kiki, piling some daal onto her roti bread, 'I've watched you two together and he is besotted with you – there's no way he's walking out on you.'

'No way,' added Kate emphatically. 'You've built a wonderful life together – and one day perhaps you'll enjoy all of the freedom that comes with not having children.'

'That's what he says,' I said, wiping away my tears. 'It's just we're not even married and so in theory he could just up sticks and walk.'

'Seriously, Lucy, he isn't going anywhere,' repeated Kiki, 'but don't take my word for it, talk to him. When is he back?'

'Tomorrow,' I said, blowing my nose.

'Well, we're on the end of the phone if you need to talk,' said Kiki, 'but I know it's going to be fine.'

I nodded that I would and began to eat, relieved that Kate was changing the subject. She was as stressed as ever – today had been the first of a series of extra days she'd be putting in at work, covering for a man on sick leave, and she'd already realised she'd taken on too much, especially as she was running the third in a series of workshops at The Lotus Room that Saturday.

On the upside the trip to Ibiza was booked; she and Will were leaving the following week for a fortnight. 'At this stage we're looking at all the options – we might join the community I told you about but we're also looking at building our own eco-friendly house – maybe Kevin McCloud will come and do a *Grand Designs* on it. We want to have a self-sufficient smallholding – and I could teach, but obviously it's a big step and we're just going to go and weigh up the options, we might also do a bit of clubbing when we're there.'

Kiki wanted to tell us about a new man she'd met, an artist who lived quite near my mum in north Norfolk. She'd chanced upon him in his seaside gallery and they'd struck up a conversation. 'Are you an artist too?' he'd asked her. Flattered, she'd suggested a coffee and they'd soon established that they had grown up together only roads apart, that their mothers knew each other and that he shared her love of film noir. They'd talked for hours so she'd taken things to the next level and invited him to her house for dinner. 'It was *such* a disappointment,' she told us, 'I cooked a really yummy curry, which wasn't well received, then he shoved my cats off the sofa and then he practically did the same thing to my son.'

I'd met her son for the first time a few weeks before – she'd brought him along to one of our retail and spiritual grooming sessions in John Lewis's recently opened espresso bar – he sat so sweetly beside me, sipping his juice and showing me *The Mighty Boosh* and *Life on Mars* on his iPod, that I'd named him the Divine Child.

'I wouldn't trust a man who didn't like kids,' said Kate.

'Or cats,' I added.

'Well, never mind, he's *a* man, but he's not *my* man,' concluded Kiki emphatically.

'Most definitely a case of "the wrong trousers",' said Kate firmly.

'Did he make any moves?' I asked, always interested in the detail.

'Nope – he left to drive back to north Norfolk. I went to bed early and curled up with the Divine Child, the cats and a cuppa and it was brilliant.'

The next morning I had my eighth and final session with the Mad Professor. I told him my FSH score and he seemed genuinely disappointed for me; his whole body seemed to sag into his feet.

I couldn't help wondering, given the way the numbers had gone, whether I'd done the right thing by having acupuncture: had it actually damaged my chances of conceiving? After my first session my period had come two weeks early – I'd thought it was stimulating my hormones but maybe it was upsetting them.

'The difficulty is that we just don't know what would have happened if you'd had no acupuncture,' he said thoughtfully, 'would your FSH have been four, or 254?'

He was right of course. I sat on the couch and concentrated on the gently glowing fish tank as he took the pin out of my ear. I found myself blinking back more tears – I'd worn it since the beginning of January, it had become a little talisman of my intention, taking it out felt like the end of all hope.

I went home to find David had arrived early – he was sitting in the kitchen with Tony the Tiler. I must admit to wishing that Tony wasn't there – I'd waited four long days for a hug from my man, but Tony was a lovely man who'd done a great job for us and so I made us some more tea and sat and listened patiently as he told us, with great pride, that his oldest son, who'd turned down a place at UEA because he'd spotted a mistake in the tutor's calculations at interview, had just accepted a place at Portsmouth reading Maths and Law. His younger son, in sixth form on a Talented and Gifted programme, had already turned down Cambridge.

As soon as Tony went upstairs to tile the bathroom floor I found myself sobbing in David's arms. 'I would've been happy with a Supremely Untalented and Ungifted child,' I wailed.

'I know, my love, I just wish there was something I could do,' he said, kissing my cheek.

'I can't help worrying that you're going to leave me for a younger model,' I said, rushing the words out, embarrassed to be confessing the thought.

'No, Babe,' he said firmly, folding me into his arms. 'I'd love children but I love you much more. I'm here to stay.'

'I just wish that we'd found each other sooner,' I said mournfully.

'Who knows what would've happened if we'd met in our twenties?' replied David. 'I don't know – would we have fallen in love? We were very different people then.'

David was right. He was working in fashion on the King's Road by day and his nights were spent in L'Equipe Anglaise. At twenty-five I was walking round the agency in shoulder-padded bouclé wool suits pretending to be Paula Hamilton in that Golf ad. I wouldn't have had time to get to the club; I would've been too busy running acetates through the photocopier in preparation for the following day's meeting.

David whisked me into Norwich – he thought some retail therapy would cheer me up, but looking in the mirror of Tosho's changing rooms I saw a woman I hardly recognised. As I pondered the potential benefits of Restalyne and Botox I realised that I was dealing with a double whammy – being too old for kids meant I was entering middle age. Desmond Morris, the anthropologist I'd worked with back in the Advertising Years, had told me that the reason youth is such a highly prized human driver is because it signifies health and fertility – being young means you are fertile, therefore being infertile means you are no longer young.

What to do? I didn't want to go under the knife and I didn't like the idea of Botox either, despite the growing rumour that a number of yoga teachers now owed their youthful vitality more to regular injections rather than their yoga practice. For the first time ever I left Tosho empty-handed.

David mistook the lack of shopping bags for a newly found self-discipline and offered to buy me dinner as a congratulatory treat. I accepted and spent the next two hours doing nothing but snap at him. I was scratchy and impatient, flat and joyless. Nothing he could do or say could make it better. He told me that he couldn't mourn the loss of something he'd never had and that he felt blessed with or without children. While I understood this argument rationally, emotionally it did nothing for me.

Returning home, comfortably reinstalled at our kitchen table, I realised that no small measure of anger had replaced the tears. I was angry with anyone who abused children – the uncle who kept his niece imprisoned under the bed, the father who locked up his daughter in a cellar and, less dramatically but closer to home, the women who slapped their children in the street. I was angry with the government – why hadn't there been a Central Office of Information publicity campaign on the subject of increasing age and decreasing fertility? Why didn't they make it clear that fertility has little to do with keeping healthy? Why didn't I know that I was born with a set number of eggs that couldn't be altered – no matter how low in fat my diet or how often I did yoga? Why didn't the government offer all women the chance to have an antral follicle ultrasound test to establish how many fertile years they'd got left? If they could spend millions on a campaign to persuade the middle-aged middle classes to curb their enthusiasm for alcohol then surely they could push a few pounds the way of young women living in blissful ignorance of their ticking biological clock – of the egg and womb race in which they were unknowingly taking part? But most of all I was angry with myself.

I gave it my best try but even I had to concede that it wasn't the government's fault that I'd left it too late to have children, it wasn't the ad agencies' fault for keeping me in the office during my child-bearing years, it wasn't the tobacco companies' fault for selling me the cigarettes that I smoked like the proverbial trooper in my twenties. I had no one to blame but myself – I never stopped to think about the bigger picture, I didn't have a life plan, hell, I didn't have a plan beyond what my secretary scheduled in my diary. Life was about working manically, emerging like a rabbit from a warren on a Saturday and indulging in a frenzy of spending in designer clothes shops. There were bigger flats, bigger salaries, bigger promotions, but I never stopped to ask myself what I would think important if I got knocked down by the number 14 bus. The idea of prioritising finding a man would've seemed so old-fashioned – I was self-important and didn't want to put myself second to anyone. When I was thirty-six Nikki, my endlessly thoughtful stepmother, had suggested that I freeze my eggs and give myself the chance of 'an ice baby' but I didn't want to do that. I stuck my head in the sand and convinced myself that if I was fit and healthy I would stand a good chance of conceiving. I didn't want to know that fertility rates fall off a cliff, that IVF can't help most women over forty, that a significant number of the babies born to older birds have egg donation to thank for it. Like that famous phrase from *A Few Good Men* I couldn't handle the truth, so I hid from it.

David sat and listened and urged me to accept these feelings and to acknowledge the loss. 'Let the experience be your teacher, my babe,' he said, gently. 'What can you learn from all of this? Do you think you might have an issue around acceptance?'

Although initially resistant, on reflection I had to admit that acceptance and I had been strangers for a long time. The experts' statistics had been pretty clear. Did I listen? Did I hell! I got an FSH reading of forty-seven and what did I do? Try to score more fertility treatments.

Granted, not accepting people's so-called words of wisdom had often served me well – the headmaster who thought I'd be lucky to get a job selling perfume, the relation who told me to get some typing skills so that 'I'd always have something to fall back on', the industry 'expert' who warned I'd never get a publishing contract because 'these days it's all about celebrity'. However, there *was* an important distinction here; when it was a question of controlling outcomes by working harder, by having more determination, by being more focused, non-acceptance was fine, but pursuing conception with any more determination or focus wasn't any more likely to result in a baby. In fact the reverse might well have been true. It was too late and that was that.

David and I discussed potential courses of action. Were there other ways in which we could parent? What about adoption? Thanks to the glowing endorsement of Brangelina, Madonna and Sheryl Crow an adopted baby was very much the 'must have' of our times; if I'd been in charge of developing a campaign for adoption I couldn't have hoped for more effective PR. I might have been able to put up with the years of waiting, the years of searching and the complete lack of a guaranteed outcome but given David's age we would only be offered children over five years old and we really wanted a baby, worried that an older child might be too emotionally damaged for us to make a difference. I guess we both believed in the old saying 'give me the child till the age of seven and I will give you the man'. It was an issue for both of us which was compounded by the rarity of adoption in Indian culture, a country in which blood ties determine everything from marriage prospects to career potential.

What about surrogacy? I quite fancied being the ex-supermodel Cheryl Tiegs who was fifty-two when she and then husband Rod Stryker used a surrogate to carry their child. I think David quite fancied being her partner Rod Stryker, the yoga teacher made rich by his self-styled 'supreme' ParaYoga. We would've gone to the Indian Centre for Reproductive Outsourcing and gladly spent £15,000 on an all-inclusive package incorporating fertilisation procedures, accommodation and plane tickets – if only my problem could have been solved by a rent-a-womb service.

We went for a walk around the gardens at South Walsham's Fairhaven Lake – it sounded like an old people's home, and to all intents and purposes it was. We followed the geriatrics seeking peace amongst the primroses, bluebells and rhododendron bushes – it seemed a fitting place to discuss what to do about my prehistoric eggs. The conversation returned to the virtues of egg donation.

Clearly there were some significant upsides, not the least of which was that it offered women of my age five times the chance of success offered by standard IVF. Egg donation also seemed to promise a break with tradition, a getting away from the old ways, the opportunity to participate in a brave new world. There was something thrilling about the prospect of becoming a fertility revolutionary – the Che Guevara of wombs. I imagined myself as a freedom fighter liberating myself and other women from the dictatorship of age, redefining motherhood. As Gabriele's friend had said, 'the key to being a mother is carrying, not conceiving'. I was sure she had a point. One of the fertility clinic nurses talked about a new phenomenon called 'Embryo Imprinting', which, if I understood her correctly, meant that there was some evidence that the baby took on the genetic material of the pregnant woman, whether or not she was the biological mother.

I also liked the idea of being as old as the woman whose eggs you receive and, as we sat watching a little boat plying the Fairhaven Lake, David played around with the idea of choosing the egg donor. I told him about some websites I'd found which required their donors to be young, beautiful, healthy and intelligent. Signing up with 'Exceptional Donors' or 'Ron's Angels' would cost us between $15,000 and $150,000 – depending on the donor's relative youth, beauty, health and intelligence.

'The problem is that current performance is no guarantee of future potential,' I mused, 'our investment's looks, health and intelligence could go down as well as up.'

David agreed – we both knew of gorgeous mothers with less blessed daughters.

'We could go by country,' joked David, 'buy some Jewish Italian eggs – they'd have smarts *and* style. Or how about some Swedish eggs? Or maybe Russian – some of those birds are really cute.'

David was, by his own account, very well behaved as a young man. Perhaps he saw this as his chance to mess around with impunity.

'I think I'll cut out the middle woman and let you get on with it,' I said briskly. 'Yes, why don't I stick someone else's genetic material in my womb, and why not mix it up with my future husband's genes? No problem!' I folded my arms and stared at the lake. Invisible steam poured forth from my ears.

'It's okay, Babe, I'm just kidding.' He put his arm round me and pulled me towards him. 'It's taken me a very long time to find you – I only want your genes and that's it.'

I also had an issue with the anonymous genetic material – although I could see its advantages – to be honest I would have been glad to have a child with a chance of a chin.

The other problem I kept coming back to was that egg donation came with a ticket to a moral maze of issues around telling and not telling; I only knew of one person who'd gone public on the issue and there seemed, in all likelihood, to be plenty of others who'd been economical with the truth. It wasn't surprising really; according to a survey by a Scottish hospital only fifteen per cent of fertile women were likely to 'approve' of a child created by egg donation. But if we didn't tell and there was a genetic problem, then what would we do? What if the child needed a blood transfusion? What reasons could we possibly come up with for not wanting to donate our blood or organs? Would we have to pretend to be Jehovah's Witnesses? I could see the *ER* story-line now, and sadly I didn't think George Clooney would be the doctor to counsel us.

*

And so came the dark day when I sat down and accepted that I would never know what it was to be a mother, biological or otherwise. I accepted that I wouldn't know what it would feel like to feed my baby, to watch his first steps, to hear about his first love. I had lost him and I had lost myself as a mother, and it was a loss that threatened to stretch out forever, if I let it – marking birthdays, weddings and funerals by its absence. I accepted and I cried, and I accepted and cried some more and to my surprise there was relief in those tears – hitting the bottom meant that there was nowhere further to fall. And eventually I stopped crying because even at the bottom of the well I could see a chink of light above me, a realisation that this loss didn't have to stretch out forever, didn't need to dictate my future. That I was blessed with or without children and that the experience could indeed, as David had suggested, be my teacher. I'd already understood that acceptance and I needed to get to know each other, what else I had to learn was not yet entirely clear, but for now I was content to know that one day, sooner or later, I would find out. As it turned out I wouldn't have to wait too long.

The only hard thing remaining was to tell my family that we wouldn't be having children. But how? How could I tell them that they weren't going to be grandparents on my watch? I felt so ashamed I didn't think I was physically capable of uttering the words.

But utter them I must. My two mums cried, telling me 'you'd have been a wonderful mother'. My two dads were full of practical solutions. Had we considered all of our options? Who had we talked to? Had we been in touch with the best clinics? I told Yvonne, David's mother, how sorry I was not to be able to play my part in carrying on the family line, privately offering up thanks for the five grandchildren David's brothers had already given her. She made tea and fed me several of Cynthia's just-baked samosas and gave me a hug that heated my entire body as effectively as our wood burner. In that moment I realised that there was no need to return ever again to the backwaters of Kerala, to queue for hours, with thousands of others, in order to be embraced by Amma, the woman who hugged for a living. I had my very own Hugging Mother and she lived in W10. She may not have whispered 'Durga, Durga, Durga' into my ear in an urgent, loud and ferociously hot whisper but she didn't need to say anything. I knew that my Hugging Mother loved me, with or without children.

16

'Namaste Norfolk'

I was keen to move on, I didn't want my fertility, or the lack thereof, to be the all-consuming focal point of my life anymore. I wasn't sure what I wanted to be the focal point, so in lieu of doing anything hasty I took a bit of time just to be, keeping myself busy with familiar routines. I took advantage of the spring sun and the easterly winds that whipped round the corners of the house to wash, mop and dust. I think it would be fair to say that there wasn't a cleaner house in Norfolk than the farmhouse that April.

When I wasn't washing or cleaning I was finding peace in the wild things; summer came early that year; the glorious Technicolor fields were bright with rapeseed, like paint-brushes dipped in yellow. Set against the blue skies, they looked like the primary colours of a child's picture book. I followed the becalmed waters of the River Waveney as it meandered towards Beccles, dandelions, marigolds and apple blossom lined the tracks, the hedgerows full of cow parsley. I breathed in the warm air scented by pollen, the sweet scent of the fruit orchards, taking refuge from the occasional rainstorm in the woods, scattering pheasants, wood pigeons and hares with every step.

When I wasn't washing or cleaning or walking I was

gardening; sharpening the grass borders with an innovative technique that required me to jump wholeheartedly on the edger, using my entire body weight to plunge it into the ground. Slightly less energetically I planted daffodils, restocked the herb garden and replanted the beds outside the front door.

When I wasn't washing or cleaning or walking or gardening I was hanging out with The Bad Ladies at yoga. I was relieved to see Kate return from Ibiza honey brown and in great shape. She'd only been away a couple of weeks but I'd really missed her, and her teaching. It was good to be back at the Quaker Meeting House, to walk past the blackboard directing 'Knit and Knatter' participants to the right, s(w)ingers straight ahead and yoga practitioners up the stairs. It was good to be back in our yoga sanctuary in the gables of the seventeenth-century house, to practise hip openers, reclining twists and backbends as the s(w)ingers rehearsed Gilbert and Sullivan's *HMS Pinafore* down below. And it was good to catch up after the class with my fellow students. Our baker was writing a weekly column for the local paper, the sprightly sixty-something was planning a trip to India with her charity, the nut-brown mum's tan reaped the benefit of days on Great Yarmouth beach with her kids, and the two teenagers had exams but managed to maintain an air of yogified bliss at all times, seemingly unfazed by the demands of their studies. But there was one woman I wanted to catch up with more than any other. Finally the door banged shut and I found myself alone with Kate.

I seized my opportunity. 'So what about Ibiza? Are you moving there?' I asked nervously.

'No,' came the welcome reply, 'it's not for us – we

realised that we wanted to stay in England, that our family and friends are what's really important.'

I resisted the urge to jump up and down on the spot, I think.

'So you're staying in Harleston?' I asked enthusiastically.

'There's no easy way to say this,' said Kate carefully, 'so I'll just come straight out with it.' She cleared her throat and looked me directly in the eye. 'We're selling the house and we're moving north of Norwich.'

'But you'll have to start all over again with your classes,' I protested. 'And your husband will have to find a new job.'

'That's okay – we don't mind starting over. I'll be giving everyone here in Beccles a month's notice – just as soon as we have a completion date on the house.'

'It's already on the market?'

'Yes, it's under offer.'

There was a pause.

'I thought you liked Harleston,' I countered, 'it's so pretty, why would you move to north Norfolk?'

'Harleston is quite busy…'

'Busy? It's got a tiny high street and its biggest shop is the deli…'

'I know, but it's still a town and we'd really like to be in the middle of nowhere. I miss the rural life,' she sighed, 'I grew up in a tiny hamlet and I want to feel that sense of space again, to be able to walk out the back door with the dogs, to not have to put them on a lead.'

'But you told me you couldn't wait to get out when you turned eighteen.'

'Things change, don't they? I'm not eighteen anymore.'

'So where will you live?'

'My aunt's found us a place that's near her – it's got some land so we can be totally self-sufficient... perhaps we'll set up our version of the Ibiza commune there.'

Finally understanding that I was on a losing wicket I gave up. 'I *am* pleased for you,' I said, 'it's what you want. It's just that I'll really miss you.'

She gave me a much stronger hug than you would imagine her slender frame would allow. 'I'm thinking of coming back to Beccles to do the occasional workshop, and of course, you can come and stay with us and we can go for walks with the dogs – it'll give you a chance to see a different part of Norfolk.'

'Okay,' I said, busying myself with rolling up my yoga mat, 'that would be great,' trying to convince myself that it would be.

Walking back to the car it seemed to me that I needed to pay another visit to my new friend acceptance.

Kiki had been raving about Claire Missingham for months, sending out 'Oh My Goddess' entitled emails promoting her to The Lotus Room crowd and telling me, 'She's the real deal, Lucy, a north London yoga goddess after your own heart.' An ex-dancer and choreographer, she did indeed have all the credentials of a modern-day yoga goddess; a mystical birth to Sufi parents who gave her the spiritual name 'Habiba', a signature yoga clothing collection and a best-selling DVD filmed on location in Marrakech. She'd made several appearances on the cover of *Yoga Journal* in which she modelled picture-perfect poses, she'd been featured in *Grazia*, *Vogue* and *Conde Nast Traveller*, she had a regular slot on cable TV's Body in Balance channel, a list of MySpace friends that included Sting, Gandhi and Deepak Chopra, a regular teaching gig at Triyoga and a packed schedule of national and international appearances.

Walking into The Lotus Room that morning I was feeling more than a little cynical. Surely someone with such strong commercial instincts couldn't really be a spiritual leader? Her clothes didn't do anything to persuade me otherwise. She was clad head to foot in her signature Sushumna clothing range – orange trousers and top with a matching grey hoodie. Bronze drop lotus earrings brought out the amber in her eyes, eyes flecked with green and yellow. The girl was the spitting image of the actress Heather Graham; her pale lineless skin translucent in the morning light, her face a delicate oval shape with a high forehead and pretty nose framed by strawberry blonde tresses that tumbled luxuriously to the bottom of her shoulder blades.

Kiki sidled up to me. 'Lucy,' she said in hushed tones, 'I thought I'd better let you know that Claire is three months pregnant. You can see her baby bump if you look closely, but I thought you might be a bit sensitive on the subject and I just wanted you to be prepared.'

Bloody great. Not only was she absolutely gorgeous, perfectly formed and the daughter of Sufis, she was also pregnant. Oh well, onwards and downwards; I could only hope that the 'Chakra Vinyasa' workshop, her signature practice, would function as advertised and lead me away from jealousy and towards 'my Spirit and highest potential'.

I walked into the practice room to find Claire sitting at her harmonium playing soothing harmonies. There were sixteen mats, arranged in two vertical rows so that we faced each other. I settled myself for comfort next to Kate and opposite Kiki.

Claire bowed her head. 'Namaste Norfolk,' she said, gently pulsating back and forth.

We bowed and said 'Namaste' in return, thereby promising that the spirit in each of us would respect the spirit in each other.

'I'd ask you all to introduce yourselves but as this is Norfolk you probably all know each other already,' she joked.

Us Bad Ladies smiled at each other in silent acknowledgement.

'This master class will show you how to use your vinyasa practice to clear the chakras and build your life force. If you get any niggles I'd recommend using China Gel,' she said, holding up a large plastic tub. 'It's great for soothing away aches and pains and you can buy some from me at the end of the class.' It turned out to be an eye-watering twenty-five pounds a tub, which gave me a pain in a different place.

'I'd like to begin by explaining the theory of the chakras,' she said as she encouraged us to pulse in time with her harmonium harmonies. 'In the West the focus is on the physical but the chakras go beyond this – they're a way of going deeper, a way of expanding our understanding of reality that is beyond the external. Chakra means "wheel" – when these wheels are spinning freely and Sushumna *Nadi*, "the main energy channel in the body", is purified *Shakti* energy can move up the spine to re-unite with Shiva. When this happens we feel grounded, loving and creative, able to express ourselves, able to feel something spiritual, able to ascend towards a blissful, compassionate, joyful experience of life.'

She gave each of us a sheet of paper explaining the

function of the chakras. 'The lower three chakras relate to your self-image and the external world. They are where we live – keeping us grounded and creative, nurturing our sense of self-esteem. At the heart centre we begin to focus inside, and the upper three chakras relate to rising above the ego, towards our spiritual self.'

After a short meditation to ensure that we 'left our journey behind' we got on with the business of clearing our chakras, starting with the one located at the base of the spine. We visualised the colour red and chanted a so-called '*Bija* or seed mantra' to purify and heal. We stood in Mountain Pose, 'to root down and establish our earth connection'. We stood in standing splits, or as close as we could get to the splits while standing, to build stability.

We chanted another mantra to purify the good old *Svadhistana* chakra, the fertility chakra located just below the navel. We visualised orange as we performed a spiralling sequence that started with rotating lunges and ended in a squat, hands in prayer position. Claire held my legs in a clamp constructed entirely of her own legs as I rotated ever deeper away from fear, aggression and obsessive addictions and towards creativity and better relationships.

We chanted '*Ram*' and stoked the fire of *Manipura* chakra with leg raises. As we hovered above the floor in Plank pose we attempted to rise above our ego, letting go of the need to be right all the time, and doing our best to emit the radiant glow of self-esteem.

I don't know if it was Ms Missingham herself, her chakra vinyasa sequence, the energy in the room, or the yogic soundtrack of Cheb I Sabbah, Neel Dhorajiwala and Niraj Chag (which I felt sure would be available on a Missingham

Mix sometime very soon) but I suddenly realised that I was feeling fantastic. I moved effortlessly through the forward bends and shoulder stands, unlocking my heart chakra as I went, and by the time I chanted '*Ham*' to purify my throat chakra and '*Om*' to tune into my third eye, settle my nervous system and awaken my intuition, I was really in the flow.

Then the pièce de resistance: performing a headstand, while chanting a silent '*Om*' to release boundless transparent white light, energy and bliss, I experienced my first-ever **spiritual epiphany**. I couldn't believe it – I had travelled all the way round India in search of one of these; I'd cleaned the ashram toilets, I'd gone to yoga classes at four in the morning, I'd sat at the feet of Gucci'd gurus and I'd never had the faintest bite at the epiphany cherry, and yet here I was in central Norwich on a Saturday morning sucking that cherry effortlessly, and boy did it taste sweet.

Finally we broke for lunch. I could hardly wait to tell The Bad Ladies, so I told them in the queue for the loo.

'Kiki, Kate! I *am* a mother!' I splurged, hardly able to contain myself.

'Really?' asked Kiki, 'did you just find out that you're pregnant?' She was packed full of delight about to be released.

'No, I think I just had my first merger with cosmic bliss,' I said, still feeling somewhat shell-shocked. 'I just realised that not having children of my own is meaningless because *all* children are my children.'

'That's awesome, Lucy,' said Kate, her eyes misting over. 'How did you get to that thought?'

'I don't know, it just popped into my head – fully formed. I just suddenly understood that it's not about what I'm not, it's about what I am, and I'm lucky because I don't have to single out any one child as my own, instead I get to love them all equally, I can be the free-floating love person!'

'Wow, Lucy, that's quite a breakthrough,' said Kiki, giving me a big hug.

'How do you think it happened? Do you think that my Sushumna *Nadi* got purified through the work we did on our chakras? Do you think Shakti rose and was reunited with Shiva? Do you think I unfurled my Thousand Petalled Lotus?'

The Bad Ladies thought it quite possible.

'I love Claire Missingham,' I said emphatically.

What do you do when you've just unfurled your Thousand Petalled Lotus?

You go shopping.

I tried on a long red evening dress with a large number of ruffles, idly wondering if I might wear it to my own wedding. I sighed and reluctantly I put it back on the rail – I was still waiting for David's proposal.

Kate wanted to know whether we liked the dress she'd earmarked for that eco wedding she'd talked about what now felt like a lifetime ago. I thought fondly of the Dom and his green chasuble made of recycled curtains but Kate's dress was about as far away from a chasuble as it's possible for a dress to get. Having agreed that she should buy it we retired to The T Lounge, the café we'd visited after Dina's workshop at the beginning of the year.

We settled with our assortment of skinny lattes and cappuccinos, none of us were detoxing anymore. I was keen to expand on the theme of free-floating love. 'The great thing about it is that I can choose the role I have with children,' I mused, keen to get feedback on the new plan. 'I'm not limited to telling them what to eat and when to eat it – I can be like my Aunty Bernice. I loved staying with her as a child; I'd spend the morning dyeing melon seeds blue and turning them into a necklace, or making tie-dye T-shirts, then we'd go to matinee performances and finish up in The Great American Disaster for a hamburger and a Coke float.'

'You can rent my son if you like,' said Kiki helpfully.

'I'd love to,' I agreed, sipping my cappuccino thoughtfully. 'I am going to reinvent what it means to be childless – why do we have to be seen as bitter miserable spinsters who hate all children because they can't have their own? It's misogynistic crap. I *love* children and I am going to lavish as much time and attention on them as possible. Plus,' I mused, 'I get to retire to my stain-free sofa and watch uninterrupted telly when it all gets too much.'

The girls agreed that a stain-free sofa was a good place to be and we returned to The Lotus Room in high spirits.

Something had happened to the divine Ms Missingham in the lunch break – she had mutated from yoga teacher to choir master.

'When we sing we create vibrations on the roof of the mouth, where we have eighty-four meridian points. We are going to divide into threes and sing the *Bija* seed mantras in a round – it'll be really uplifting and healing and you'll free yourself of tension.'

Kiki, Kate and I formed a small cluster group; we called ourselves The Bee Jas, Norfolk's answer to the Bee Gees.

'The human voice is designed to sing, our soul is a song in our hearts that must be heard,' said Claire encouragingly.

And off we went, our threesome leading the field with a rousing rendition of '*Lam, Vam, Ram, Yam, Ham, Om.*'

Ten minutes later my Thousand Petalled Lotus had been blown away for the second time in a day.

'Next time you see me I will be with my child,' concluded Claire. 'Perhaps she will know the colours of all the chakras by then,' she joked, 'and perhaps she will be practising on a mini-mat next to me.'

I realised that I was nothing but thrilled at the prospect of welcoming a new child, a yogi baby, to this world; a baby that I would be in some small part responsible for, even if we never met, now that all children were my children. I went home and ordered a pair of orange Sushumna leggings in celebration. Kate, in a show of solidarity, ordered a pair in Tibetan Red. Kiki already had all of them in all the colours.

The following Tuesday I met up with Kiki at her class, she gave me a big hug and congratulated me for 'rocking the Claire M look' in my Sushumna leggings.

'Ooh,' said a passing man who'd just returned from an ashram in India, 'you couldn't wear those orange leggings in the ashram I went to – you'd be mistaken for a swami.'

'It's a risk I think you can take, Lucy,' said Kiki, stifling a laugh.

After the class I slipped my jeans on and Kiki changed into a black trouser suit complete with waistcoat, trilby and heels and together we headed down to Baba Ghanoush, where we settled into a candlelit corner table and ordered a bottle of Pinot Grigio and a fish stew. Soon we were giggling about imposter swamis and the woman we'd talked to after class, a pole dancer at Spearmint Rhino who claimed to consume two bottles of Pinot Grigio and a tub of Baskin Robbins a night and wondered why she'd been hospitalised with blood poisoning. She also claimed one of Norwich's yoga teachers was an ex-pole dancer from Lowestoft so we weren't sure she was entirely reliable, but as we could see that there was a certain overlap of skills between the two careers, we didn't dismiss the idea entirely… in fact, we spent several minutes considering the prospects of 'Pologa' – a fusion between pole dancing and yoga – and wondered why us Bad Ladies hadn't thought of it before.

Kiki had an announcement to make. She'd met a new man on *Guardian* Soulmates. They'd had two dates so far and he'd already taken his profile down, suggesting that he was serious about her. They'd met at Liverpool Street station the previous week and spent two hours talking as if they were old friends. He'd driven up to Cambridge the following Saturday to meet her after a yoga workshop she was running – they'd had their first snog on the steps of her B&B and then he'd left, driving all the way back to London without imposing himself upon her.

'He totally gets me, Lucy,' said Kiki with some degree of wonderment.

'That's brilliant, Kiki,' I said, delighted by this news. 'Occupation?'

'He's a cameraman, he does lots of ads and films…'

'Star sign?'

'His sun is in Gemini and his moon is in Leo and he's done our synastry, to find out if we are a good astrological match, and we are.'

'Relationship history?'

'His ex was a New York Jew so he is obviously used to strong women.'

There then followed a spate of texts from Mr Gemini

which culminated in a picture of a blossom, the accompanying message suggesting this should be interpreted as a metaphor for the state of their relationship.

There seemed to be only one downside to this man: he was forty-nine years old and lived in a rented flat-share in Islington. We workshopped what this might indicate about his personality; did he lack ambition? Was he the first N1 swami – eschewing material possessions in favour of communal living? He hadn't displayed a fondness for orange but then again Kiki had only seen him twice. We agreed that we shouldn't rush to conclusions.

'Does he want children, Kiki?'

'No, he already has a daughter, she's in her twenties. Just as well really, because my parenting days are done. You know, Lucy, I think I'm menopausal – I'm putting on weight round my middle, I'm even getting hot flushes.'

'Maybe it's just the heat, Kiki, it has been unseasonably warm recently.'

'Maybe, but I'm also all over the shop hormonally and emotionally.'

'I know the feeling,' I said ruefully.

She paused, reaching across the table to take my hand. 'I wish I were younger and could donate my eggs to you. Sadly it looks as if mine are all shot to shit too.'

I thanked her – a Russian Polish Jew mixed with an Indian Pakistani Catholic – now that would have been an interesting mix.

'Perhaps you could go and get another hug from the Hugging Mother of Kerala, make a wish, ask for some children, see what happens,' she suggested.

I'd been down that road before and I wasn't going down

it again, and anyway, I now had my own Hugging Mother and she only lived a couple of hours away.

'It's funny,' said Kiki reflectively, 'I had my daughters at twenty-four because I didn't know what else to do with my life. I'm really glad that I have them, and my son, they're beautiful and I know that I did a good job, but I was often bored wheeling them around the park and I know I missed out on pursuing my own creativity. Part of me wants what you've got – a successful career in advertising behind you, a writing career ahead of you, a gorgeous man who knows his own mind and will never be a sponge, a lovely house, but then again,' and here was the deal breaker, 'I have children.'

There was no arguing with that – none of us gets everything in this world, and I knew that I had been blessed with more than most.

'It's tough, isn't it,' I replied, sipping my glass of wine thoughtfully. 'When I look back on it I wonder what I might have done differently. I could never have been one of those women who sees marrying a rich man as the only business plan they'll ever need – I was brought up to make my own way in the world, not to rely on a man financially, and though there were notable truths, I generally got a lot of satisfaction from my work. Part of me wishes I'd just found a sperm donor and got on with it in my twenties – but I always thought the point of having a child was doing it with the person you love – seeing how your genes turned out when they were mixed up. Plus I would've been a single mother and how much fun would that have been for the child, or me? Perhaps I couldn't have done it any other way – how it was, well, that's exactly how it needed to be – it may have taken me a while but I found the right man eventually. I had to be true to myself – and I just have to accept that we don't always get everything we want.'

'Perhaps it's helpful to think about it from a yoga perspective?' suggested Kiki. 'It teaches us to follow the natural seasons of life – to accept that our twenties are a more yin, a more feminine, time – I think we should honour that.'

'That's right, exactly right,' I said with excitement, 'I live in the country, I watch the seasons pass, the farmers hard at work, and I've only just got it! We have to accept that there is a natural time for growing, as there is a natural time for reaping what we sow. Until someone comes up with a reliable egg-freezing programme that all women can access in their twenties we have to abide by nature's rules.'

'As we get older we can develop more yang, more male energy but I think it's sad when we see young female yogis with lean masculine bodies hellbent on muscular strength.'

I agreed, the yoga calendars were full of young women with zero body fat and grim expressions on their faces, balancing on just one of their sinewy arms – sure, they didn't need to model themselves on Boticelli's *Venus* but certainly there could be more celebration of the natural contours of the female body.

'Yoga also teaches us to honour the *who*, and focus less on the *what*,' continued Kiki. 'In our twenties there is still way too much emphasis on *what* we are – *what* we have achieved and *what* we own – when it should be about *who* we are and *who* we are becoming.'

That was also true – if I'd better understood myself in my twenties, understood the *who* of me rather than focusing on the *what* of me – *what* I was achieving, *what* I owned –

then perhaps it wouldn't have taken me so long to find myself, or a man.

'These days even babies are in danger of becoming a *what* rather than a *who* – treated as if they are objects, the latest designer accessory,' said Kiki, sipping her Pinot Grigio. 'I go to London and see all these babies hanging out in designer four-by-four prams, children going to the right nurseries, wearing dresses from Elias and Grace because that's where Gwen Stefani does her kids' shopping…'

I interrupted Kiki to tell her some of Gabriele's stories concerning the competitive world of north London parenting. 'David says kids nowadays are born with a job description; to be arm candy for their parents when they're born, to enable their parents to show off their achievements as they grow, and to look after their parents when they're old.'

'Babies aren't our possessions, they don't define us and we can't live our lives through them – our mothers' generation tried that and it didn't work,' sighed Kiki. 'It's the same with everything in the West – we identify with our body, our mind's thoughts, our house, our car, our boyfriend, our husband, our children – we say "this is me" but you and I know that it's not. Yoga aims to liberate us from all that – to see that we are, to coin a phrase, "just a drop in the pool of cosmic bliss that is the universe".'

'My spiritual epiphany at The Lotus Room was about being a universal mother – a mother to children everywhere,' I added, 'what you're saying is an extension of that. The other day I found a Kahlil Gibran poem that sums this up; now, how does it go? "Your children are not your children … though they are with you they don't belong to you…

255

they're part of life's longing for itself, they came through you but not from you", or something like that.'

'Exactly,' said Kiki, exuding beatitude.

Kate and I met again the following Tuesday at Kiki's class. Afterwards the three of us walked through the centre of Norwich to Prince of Wales Road, where girls wearing belts as skirts and men with hope in their eyes went to drink. My miniskirt was somewhat longer, covering my entire bottom, and my top also afforded more than average coverage – draping my cleavage in layers of turquoise silk jersey. Kiki wore a black bat-winged jumper, satin pencil skirt, opaque tights and black suede Louis XIV shoes with huge black ribbons, Kate modelled a floaty pale yellow summer dress. We were destined for Sing Sing to celebrate Kiki's birthday.

I'd never been to a proper karaoke club before and initially found the long thin room and padded walls a little intimidating, even if they were made of white leatherette, but, aided by a couple of lemon meringue Martinis, I was soon bouncing off the walls with the best of them. It turned out that Kate had a voice that could actually carry songs by Alanis Morissette, Joni Mitchell and Tracy Chapman. Kiki and I found our level with 'Club Tropicana' and 'Dancing Queen' but it was the group anthems that I loved best – Jack Johnson's 'Better When We're Together', Queen's 'Don't Stop Me Now', Chaka Khan's 'I'm Every Woman' and the Moulin Rouge version of 'Lady Marmalade', in which we got in touch with our Bad Lady alter egos – Christina Aguilera (Kiki), Mya (Kate), Pink (me).

By the end of the evening I was hoarse and deaf and rapidly approaching my second **spiritual epiphany** in the space of a fortnight. Singing those anthems with my fellow Bad Ladies I felt a blissful cosmic merger with women everywhere. I got the bus home singing 'I'm Every Woman' to an empty top deck and, as I sat in my kitchen consuming tea and toast in an effort to recalibrate my post-karaoke high, it struck me that in this age of city living, of independent women living separate lives, it would help us if we could see ourselves as a community who collectively can have it all. If we could only aspire to view other women as manifestations of ourselves, of other choices we could make – to have children, to not have children, to succeed in business, to teach yoga, to write – then we could achieve anything and everything and, because of this, we would support each other in these choices. Those of us without children would stop bitching about maternity leave for mothers, and maybe those mothers on maternity leave would see that it was also important for the childfree to get some time off for their creative endeavours; we could call them 'Second Chakra Career Breaks' and campaign for every company to provide them.

Spiritual epiphany number three came to me in a rather different setting – the gardens of Somerleyton Hall. David and I spent one Sunday afternoon in early May driving through the sprawling villages of Toft Monks, Haddiscoe and Herringfleet, emerging to a village green around which were arranged some thirty-five identical thatched and red-timbered houses, built by Sir Morton Peto, a benevolent multi-millionaire, to show 'rare attention to the comfort and morality of peasant families'.

Peto started life as a brickie's assistant and rose to make millions constructing Nelson's Column, the Houses of

Parliament and the Russian railway – by the age of thirty he'd accrued enough money to buy Somerleyton Hall, parts of which were now open to the public. We took a tour of the house, wearing elasticised blue plastic over our shoes to protect the Crossley carpets – an area of particular sensitivity given that the current owner's great-grandfather, a Yorkshire man, had bought the house with the fortune he'd made in that business. We wandered amongst the peculiar assembly of stately memorabilia – a jar of jellybeans given by Ronald Reagan to the current Lord Somerleyton when he was Master of our Horses, a jockey's stool used to weigh the guests on arrival and departure to make sure they'd enjoyed the generosity of the house enough to put on a few pounds, two towering yellow and moth-eaten polar bears on their hind legs. There were pictures of Hugh Crossley, the only son and heir, competing in the New York marathon, and there was a painting of a more relaxed Hugh in pink shirt and jeans, against a stylised backdrop of trees. He was rather handsome in a Hugh Grant sort of way, and I had him in mind for Kiki or Andrea, until I learned that he'd just got engaged. Damn it.

While the house was a long way from its glory days the gardens had probably never looked better. The grass was immaculately rolled and smooth as velvet, clematis climbed the walls of the Paxton glasshouses, pink rhododendrons and azaleas struggled to contain themselves. As David and I wandered beneath the canopies of seventy-foot-high eucalyptus trees and cedars, wondering if the sunshine was about to turn to snow as forecast, we talked about the choices we make, choices that become turning point chapters in the story of our lives.

'I think that we've created a problem for ourselves by creating a notion of "the right time" to have a child,' said David. 'We're always waiting for the right partner, the right house, the right job... we don't want to make choices that might be wrong and that exclude other options, so "the right time" to have a child goes on getting delayed.'

'It's as if we've grown up in the era of multiple choice and we don't want to be limited to ticking one box,' I said, 'so we don't tick any boxes, we just go on keeping our options open until, ironically, we have no options left. You know I'm not even sure the women who did tick boxes were any luckier, really. *Having* it all seems, more often than not, to mean *doing* it all; my friends, women who work and have children, are often exhausted and always beating themselves up for what they haven't done.'

I was reminded of the conversation I had with Kiki at Baba Ghanoush; yoga teaches us to honour *who* we are being, not *what* we have. 'Why feel guilty for not living up to some impossible standard when you could become a standard bearer for the way you want to live, the way you want to work – in the end it's the freedom to be who we are, to enjoy people and our relationship with those people that makes us happy, and if that means the kids go to school without brushing their teeth or Mum doesn't get to the gym three times a week, then so what?'

'You know, Babe, I'm glad we're in the position we are,' said David, slinging his arm around me and pulling me closer. 'Our lives are simple – we don't have to struggle with "having it all", we are free to indulge ourselves and enjoy all of our nephews and nieces when we want to, but I will tell them, when the time comes, to get clear – to make informed choices at a time in their life when they have real choices – and if a niece of mine has found her man and is certain that she wants children I will tell her to go ahead and have them, and if she hasn't found the man but thinks there is a chance she will want children later, I will tell her to freeze her eggs.'

I agreed with him. 'I wish with all my heart that I had frozen my eggs but it just wasn't a talked-about option twenty-five years ago.'

What to do? I could be resentful of Kiki and her children, of Gabriele and Poppy, of Kate and the Angel Wah Wah and the possibility of children they had, to be bitter towards anyone who had what I didn't, but it didn't interest me.

'The only thing I can do now is to choose who I am being, choose my response, and I am *not* going to be a victim to this,' I said firmly, making my announcement to a statue of Mercury surrounded by pampas grass.

'You're bigger than that, Babe,' said David, kissing me on the cheek in a rare public display of affection. 'You could make your life about how we couldn't have kids, or you could make your life about who you *are* and what you *can* bring to the world.'

'Something tells me it may not be easy,' I admitted; 'it will probably require lots of effort and self-discipline, but as Pattabhi Jois says to his yoga students, "practise and all is coming".'

I'd been to Mysore and bought the T-shirt, and it was time to start the practice, beginning right now.

'You can be inspired by all the brilliant women who didn't have children, women who've taken all that energy and passion and done the most amazing things in their life,' suggested David.

'That's right, there is nothing of the victim in Oprah Winfrey is there? She took all that love she felt for children and put it into her Leadership Academy for Girls. What should I do, I wonder?'

'There are plenty of places to put your love, my love,' said David supportively. 'Give it some time, let it evolve. I think the important thing right now is to enjoy the freedom we've been given and get on with having the most amazing life together.'

My new resolve was tested immediately – two days later David's sister-in-law Katarina and my stepsister Victoria made their own announcements – they were both pregnant and expecting in September. I was genuinely happy for them and pleased that we would have two additions to our growing brood of nephews and nieces. When I had the inevitable wobble I mentally put on my 'practise and all is coming' T-shirt and I knew who I was again.

17

'At least she's not going commando'

It was the middle of May and spurred on by the coming of summer and a budget drained by the bottomless pit that was the farmhouse David and I took to exploring some of the holiday hotspots on Norfolk's east coast. We spent one Friday evening in Oulton Broad, the broadest of the Broads' tributaries. We walked out to the water's edge to watch the sun going down, past the teenage girls parading up and down the quay showing off honey-brown legs and the short-est of skirts, past the line of young lads smoking and fishing and checking out the girls with equal amounts of concen-tration. Standing at the end of land, the fishermen and the girls with honeyed legs behind us, a group of sleeping ducks beside us, moored up Gin Palaces and million-pound houses in front of us, it was almost possible to imagine ourselves on the French Riviera.

Bridges Wine Bar was rather more British; a gang of young women in neon-coloured satin dresses and heels were revving up for a night out – fuelled by lurid-looking cocktails they stood up one by one for their 'pap shot'; 'it's like *Heat* magazine,' one screamed. 'Or *Sex and the City*,' shouted another. Finally the ringleader wrapped her ankles, yogi-style, behind her neck, presumably for the benefit of a nearby group of neatly turned-out men with slicked-back hair.

'At least she's not going commando,' said David, calmly sipping his pint.

Our favourite stretch of water lay between Lowestoft and Southwold. We would never have found it but for Kate's tip-off. 'Just follow the narrow track all the way down until you get to the cliff edge,' she'd whispered. I wondered if, having told me, she'd have to kill me but I lived to tell the tale. We walked gingerly across the crumbling cliff tops, not far from a ledge that threatened to disappear into the sea below at any moment. Eventually the footpath dropped down towards a lake, a wildlife sanctuary that was home to more than a hundred different kinds of bird, and beyond that lay a long white beach.

We sat on the bleached and barkless remains of a fallen tree, another casualty of one of the fastest-eroding coastlines in Britain, and watched the North Sea pummel the sand into ever-tinier grains. The beach was covered in trees like this, trees that had long since lost their resemblance to living objects; the pieces of grey and white driftwood looked more like the ancient relics of a species that had died instanta-neously, mysteriously killed during a titanic extraterrestrial battle worthy of *The X-Files*.

Perched on that fallen tree, I realised that somewhere along the line, ten months after we'd been given the keys to the farmhouse, I'd finally arrived in the county; my body clock now firmly on Norfolk time. I wasn't thinking about London anymore, to be honest it felt like a different country. Yes, I was glad when London came to me; the Cappuccino

Gurus had come to stay in early May, spreading out on the lawn in their glamorous new sundresses, drinking Pinot Grigio and updating me on their latest achievements – Gabriele's soon to be finished novel, Poppy's sitting room on the cover of *Homes and Garden*, Andrea's plans to launch her organic cosmetic brand in Russia. I'd looked at my once fashionable beaded flip flops rising up out of the long grass. My toenails were a mess. When had I last had a pedicure? I was now what estate agents might term 'in need of some refurbishment', but I didn't care. It was clear that I was growing roots in Norfolk – it had exercised a secret seduction, cast a slow spell, but now I was held, as besotted as one of Casanova's mistresses, in the palm of its hand.

'Do you think Blake might've been writing about Norfolk when he wrote about England's "green and pleasant land"?' mused David as we sat in our garden one evening watching the low sun spreading long shadows across the fields. It seemed to me that this might be true, as summer opened up the landscape, unwrapping Norfolk's beneficence of space, it was possible, to coin a phrase, to 'stumble on divinity' at every turn – in the dawn chorus, in the hot dusty smell of ripening rapeseed, in the vast skies, in the fields of wheat that stretched as far as the eye could see, in the church spires that marked the edge of the horizon.

'We should have our wedding reception here,' mused David, 'the garden is looking fantastic.'

'That would be great – but aren't you getting a little ahead of yourself?' I retorted quickly. 'We aren't even engaged.' Although the summer was helping me put the failed fertility quest behind me there was still a small part of me that worried David might leave for a younger model.

When I thought about it logically there was no evidence for this, he'd been nothing short of brilliant about the whole thing, endlessly sympathetic and understanding, always by my side even when he was a hundred miles away, but still, there'd been no talk of getting married and so I'd put the thought away in a drawer, carefully wrapping it up, to be opened another time.

He reached into his jacket pocket and pulled out a small leather box, placing it gently on the table in front of me, next to my wine glass. 'Babe, I've been carrying this around ever since our FSH news, but you were so busy having spiritual epiphanies I couldn't find the right moment.'

I hardly dared breathe. Was this what I'd hoped for?

Opening the box with trembling fingers I found, nestling beneath some tissue paper, a solitaire diamond on a white gold band.

'What do you think?' asked David, looking into the far distance at a large tractor working its way up and down a field.

'Yes,' I said, my chest heaving with happiness, my eyes welling up. 'Yes.'

'Cool, Babe,' said David, finishing his glass of wine. 'Let's do it soon and do it small – I don't want any fuss.'

Absolutely fine by me.

David and I had been through a lot in the past year and we could have grown apart, the non-appearance of children might have wrecked our relationship, but instead we'd grown closer, bonded by the truth we'd spoken and the trust we'd received. Getting married would be a celebration of the distance that we'd come together, made more special because it would be done in the knowledge that the marriage wouldn't be blessed by children. I knew that David and I would have raised great kids – but I also knew that we could be great without them, and that we could make a difference to the lives of our nephews and nieces, our friends' children and all of the children we didn't yet know. In a funny way, whether or not we had children of our own didn't seem to matter anymore. We were still the same people, still throwing all of our energy into the world – and our plan was to leave it a better place.

I'd never been one of those girls who'd spent hours daydreaming about their wedding day and I had only one notion that was set in stone. The wedding reception would be held at home, on that point I was clear. I'd stood at the kitchen window on that cold February day and seen champagne in the rose garden and speeches in a marquee; being able to visualise our wedding in the garden had been one of the reasons I'd fallen in love with the farmhouse. Now, over a year later, the vision remained exactly the same, except that now I had a couple of Bad Ladies to add to the guest list.

Where did we want to get married? That seemed slightly more complicated. Although I had come to love the morning service at Our Lady of Perpetual Succour it was more because I loved the sense of community, the reminder that I was only a tiny part of something much bigger than myself and because I loved the Dom's homilies on love, life and how to live it, than because of any newly discovered religious fervour. I was, for a while, keen to get married at the registry office. This plan fell by the wayside when the clerk who registered our intentions asked if we'd like to see the room in which we would be married.

'That would be good,' we agreed.

'I'll just go and check it's okay,' she said, disappearing into the aforementioned room.

She reappeared. 'Yes, that's fine. Come in,' she said, standing in the doorway.

We walked in to find a wedding in full swing – the couple were signing the register.

We got out faster than you could say 'I will' but it still seemed to take an eternity to leave the room.

I felt absolutely terrible for interrupting their ceremony, and there was no way I was going to risk having the same thing happen to us. Plus there was something soulless about the place – the arrows on the floor guiding you through the process as if you were on a conveyor belt, the clerk who was in a hurry to get through our interview so she could get to her doctor's appointment, the tight timetable of weddings at half-hour intervals that resulted in holding pens full of nervous men and pink-suited women.

The Dom dropped in on us that evening. He was as horrified as we were.

'I will marry you,' he said firmly. 'We will do it at my church.'

'Does it matter that I'm not a Catholic?' I asked, pouring him a second glass of David's best Rioja.

'Not at all,' came the fast reply.

'Great,' said David and I in unison, realising that it was so clearly the right thing to do that neither of us could believe we'd ever considered doing anything else.

Within the hour I'd rung all the yoga girls and all, bar the Angel and Gabriele (who would be on holiday), were able to attend the wedding, to be held on the first Saturday in July – the anniversary of our move into the house.

*

The next big question was what to wear. Truth be told I had some trouble getting a clear idea of what Lucy the bride looked like; the only thing I knew was that I wouldn't be wearing the red ruffle dress I'd tried on the day of my first spiritual epiphany – I had a feeling it wouldn't go down too well with Our Lady of Perpetual Succour. I wished that I could call on Kiki but she was away for a fortnight, teaching on a yoga retreat in Italy.

I decided to spend a couple of days in London finding the dress of my dreams – I'd do it on my own, without any fuss – how hard could it be? I'd try on lots of styles and something would speak to me. I started in Harrods. The nineteen-year-old sales assistant looked at my reflection in the mirror and asked me if it was my second, or perhaps my third wedding. I spent half a day in Selfridges wandering vacantly from rail to rail, eventually I bought myself a new pair of jeans but despite a brief flirtation with the idea, even I had to admit that going Haute Gap Year on my wedding day wasn't going to be a good look. I made an appointment at a well-heeled South Molton Street store and found myself in the hands of a skinny fifty-something woman in long stockings, miniskirt and dyed blonde plaits – a look that didn't fill me with confidence. It soon became apparent that she was only pretending to be my personal stylist – dumping three evening dresses in the changing room and disappearing to make tea until I'd worked out that they all looked hideous on me and completely unlike a bride.

I rang Poppy in a panic early the next morning. Could she apply her talent for transforming interiors to my exterior? Was she available right now? Half an hour later she appeared, clutching a large coffee and the details of her favourite designers.

We started with a traditional bridal store; perhaps a long white number would make me feel the part. Poppy installed herself on a large dove-grey velvet sofa and traded her coffee for champagne. I stood in the changing rooms with my arms in the air as the sales assistant dropped one gorgeous confection after another over my head. Something happened in their transition from softly padded coat hanger to my body – perhaps it was to do with my own soft padding, but most of them did me no favours, and several of them highlighted unforeseen problems.

'At least your back is still good,' said the sales assistant brightly.

Three of the ten dresses were passable – those with the most corsetry – but the price tags ranged from £500 to £4,000, and I found it vaguely depressing to think I needed to spend such a serious amount of money to look good. I also had doubts about the appropriateness of wearing a big white dress – a line from *Sex and the City the Movie* was ringing in my ears; according to Carrie's *Vogue* editor, forty was the cutoff point for being photographed in a wedding gown. According to her, at forty-three I was well past the gown stage and, more importantly, it just didn't feel right to me. Carrie may have started out in acres of satin and taffeta Vivienne Westwood but she'd been a lot happier in the label-free ivory vintage suit that she wore when she finally clinched the deal. I felt the same way. Poppy bundled me into a taxi and fifteen minutes later I found myself in a private salon in Notting Hill.

Poppy took another glass of champagne and stationed

herself on a raspberry velvet chaise longue beneath a huge gilt mirror and chandelier. Beautiful dresses covered every available inch of wall space. And there it was: a full-length fuchsia dress made of romantic chiffon, elegant, providing coverage in all the right places, and not costing £4,000.

'It's perfect, Lucy,' said Poppy enthusiastically. 'Pink is so Indian – we can make it a Bollywood wedding; there'll be fuchsia roses everywhere, we'll use fuchsia swags in the marquee, fuchsia floor cushions in the chill-out room… and we'll get you lots of bling.'

We took lots of photos and left the dress behind for alterations.

And that should've been it – the beginning of a fairy-tale ending, and yet every time I thought about the dress I got a curious twisting feeling in my stomach. It just didn't feel right; there was something a little too covered up about it, too formal, too stiff – quite an achievement for chiffon. I decided to show the photo of me in the dress to David.

'I thought we were having an informal wedding,' he said. 'Wouldn't you prefer to wear something more glamorous, something shorter?'

If anyone knew about glamorous dresses it was Kiki. I waited for her return from the olive groves of Tuscany and together we went to London for the day. It was brilliant to see her again. Despite missing her connection because she forgot to adjust to local time, losing her yoga mat bag in a luggage mix-up, having to change rooms twice due to 1) bad drain smells and 2) general pokiness, and getting locked out of her room at six in the morning when she went to investigate a clanging sound, she'd actually had a rather fabulous time and looked every inch the tanned yoga goddess. I thought of those keenly fought poolside body fat contests at the Southern Star hotel in Mysore and knew that she would've been the clear winner.

I showed her the pink chiffon number. Thankfully they hadn't started on the alterations and said I could swap it for something else.

'What do you think?' I asked, twirling around in its many layers.

'It would be okay if you were going to the opera,' she replied, making a face.

She disappeared for a few minutes and returned with armfuls of dresses. 'How about this one?' she asked, thrusting through the curtains a sleeveless knee-length cream dress with rippling chiffon layers and elaborate bronze beading.

Why hadn't I seen it before? I suppose I'd been looking at the longer dresses with plenty of coverage, and I'd become very caught up in the idea of matching the room in my Bollywood-themed wedding.

This dress was gorgeous. I tried it on, it fitted like a dream. I felt glamorous, sophisticated, feminine and sexy. I felt perfect.

Even though we were having a small wedding we'd only given ourselves six weeks to get the whole thing organised and the arrangements took over my life. After several false starts in which the local florist refused to work with the flowers we were being given as a wedding present, the DJ we'd found in The Yellow Pages who insisted 'every wedding needs a cheese section' comprising 'The Cha Cha Slide', 'The Macarana', 'The Timewarp' and 'YMCA', and a chef who came to give us a taste of what he could do and gave us both stomach upsets, I stopped messing around and paid a visit to Lady Birkie. She sat me down in her gloriously bright and elegant sitting room with a plateful of chocolate fancies and extra-strong coffee, and once again opened her address book on our behalf. Lucky for us she'd still got all the numbers from her recent endeavours: a party for her eldest son, a parents' day at her youngest daughter's school, and canapés for a local artist's private view. I left with the names of Norfolk's finest florists, DJs and chefs.

In amongst all the arranging yoga became my lifeline – a refuge from decisions about florists, DJs and chefs. I regained my sanity with the Angel Wah Wah and Kiki at The Lotus Room and with Kate at the Quaker Meeting House, often crossing paths with the bustling Knit and Knatter brigade, for whom the knitting apparently never stopped, despite the hot weather. The Beccles S(w)ingers remained in full swing, singing their hearts out and providing us with a soundtrack somewhat at odds with the slow steady rhythms of our vinyasa flow classes.

I managed to snatch the odd hour for an update with The Bad Ladies. Kate and I went to The Swan House for some après yoga Pinot Grigio. She and Will had moved into their new home in a tiny hamlet surrounded by fields and woods.

'How are you settling in?' I asked her.

'Well, it's a bit different to living in Harleston,' she laughed, 'it's remote rural – I go to the nearest market town a few miles away and it all seems a bit too busy, and Norwich is suddenly a big city – way too intense for me! We love it though, we spent this morning with the dogs hunting for truffles in the woods; I have to tell you, I don't miss the office job one bit. I'm really enjoying reconnecting with my family and I get to spend time with Will and do things together – we've painted the house and now we're building a wood store.'

This girl didn't hang about. 'And what will be happening to the classes in Beccles?' I asked, as mildly as I could.

'I'm going to make an official announcement next week but I'll tell you now – I finish teaching my Wednesday night classes at the end of June, and meanwhile I'm trying to establish some classes a bit closer to home.'

'How far is it from Beccles to your new place?' I asked.

'About an hour.'

I'd always counted myself as something of a yoga enthusiast but even I wasn't prepared to spend an hour getting to a yoga class. I was gutted.

'We'll work something out, Lucy,' said Kate, 'perhaps I could come over to you and we could do our own practice together sometimes?'

'That would be brilliant,' I replied enthusiastically. 'We could take it in turns – I'll come to you too, we can walk your dogs and hunt for truffles together.'

'Great – and you'll see Will's polytunnel. We'll be entirely self-sufficient by this time next year and he's going to use it to grow fruit trees from cuttings which we can then sell. By the way, we're going to have a polytunnel-warming party later in the summer, will you and David come?'

I had never been to a polytunnel-warming party before but I was already looking forward to it.

Kiki invited Kate and me for dinner at her house. Over spaghetti and a bottle of Pinot Grigio in her bewitching lantern-lit garden, the kind of overgrown garden I would've imagined full of fairies as a child, she debriefed us on the status of her relationship with Mr Gemini. She was feeling flat and unexcited about their future together.

'I don't know, girls,' she said slowly, 'he gets my sense of humour and he's the perfect boyfriend in many ways but I'm not feeling it. Am I too old? Perhaps meeting someone in your forties is different.'

We agreed that it was unlikely to have quite the giddy excitement of a first love but it should still feel right, and there shouldn't be a feeling of needing to change in order to make the other person happy; there'd been some unfortunate incidences in which he'd appeared to be just a tad controlling:

'Do you really need to eat all those rice crackers just before we go for dinner?'

'Are you going to wear that top again?'

'Aren't you going to wipe the table before we eat?'

'That's outrageous,' said Kate, polishing off her glass of wine with some vigour.

'He does have *some* upsides,' Kiki conceded, 'he's very kind in some ways, and very funny, occasionally, but I don't know... my heart's just not in it,' she said glumly, staring at the lanterns glowing in the dark. 'I'd better see where he's at but to be honest I've been on my own too long to be able to tolerate being told what to eat, clean and wear.'

She met up with Mr Gemini at Cambridge train station – a halfway point for each of them – a couple of days later. I think Kiki would've loved it to work out – but perhaps she was more in love with the idea of being in love than with Mr Gemini himself. I think she'd hoped that it might turn out like one of her favourite films of the forties – in which star-crossed lovers meet on the platform with tears in their eyes, their tightly buttoned jackets heaving with suppressed emotion. They'd whisper clipped sentences in period accents as brittle as bone china and all misunderstandings would melt away, the camera panning to the magnificent train pulling out of the station, leaving the embracing couple and their suitcases shrouded in steam. No, he made further suggestions concerning her appearance and home, at which point she found it effortless to split up with him.

The sleeveless dress that I would be wearing on my wedding day might've been perfect but my arms were less so. Long before the wedding dress episode Kiki had pointed out to me that they needed some work. 'That's why your *Chaturanga* is collapsing,' she explained, 'and that's why you're finding it hard to do all the arm balances. You're a Bad Lady! Let me sort you out with a weights programme that'll give you buff arms in weeks.'

I met her at her gym; it was the first time I'd been in one since I started practising yoga ten years ago.

'It's not just for the wedding dress,' I found myself saying, 'it's for my yoga practice too – when I have strong arms I will be able to do *Chaturanga* really well, and all those arm balances.'

Kiki smiled to herself and put together a twenty-minute buff-arm programme that she guaranteed would achieve sculpted arms by W Day.

I spent the next four weeks working my deltoids, triceps and biceps through a series of increasingly heavy weights and lo and behold, after a fortnight I started to see signs of nascent muscle activity. There was an unexpected and most welcome side effect – by the time I'd finished my boobs had lifted at least two centimetres, and seemed to fill out – it was as if I'd had cosmetic surgery without the pain (well, without most of the pain) and without the expense. I would like to take this opportunity to thank Kiki for her wedding gift – it was quite the best present David received.

Kiki and I decided that my yoga practice would also benefit from stronger abs, and the W Day dress would look better – a useful side effect that was not at all the main reason for asking the Angel Wah Wah for the precise details of the *Nabhi Kriya*.

'It will really strengthen your third chakra and realign your pelvis,' explained the Angel, handing me the piece of paper, 'and my friend who did it, a mum who'd had love handles ever since she'd had children, got rid of them completely by doing the *kriya* for forty days. A City man on my teacher-training course did it and he says it's made a huge difference to his ability to communicate – he feels so much more centred and deals are landing in his lap.'

Deals landing in his lap? Could be very handy as those wedding bills were mounting up. I was in.

I enjoyed the so-called recovery position – knees to chest for five minutes – designed to eliminate gas and relax the heart, and I loved 'charging the magnetic field' which happened when I lay on my back and opened my arms out to the side while extending my legs to sixty degrees 'like a flower unfurling', but three days later my groin muscles were so tight I could hardly walk. I blamed the alternate leg lifts – no amount of 'deep powerful breathing' would carry me to the prescribed ten minutes, or even the four minutes that the Angel had suggested that I begin with. I persevered, I was fully committed to the process; I wanted wedding deals to land in my lap and for my third chakra to be strengthened and, by the way, to look lithe in my wedding dress, but a week later there was a new problem – my lower back was killing me.

Kiki had a look at my technique. 'Stop that immediately,' she advised, her brow furrowed with concern. 'Your stomach muscles aren't strong enough to do them without damaging your spine.' I was gutted – I'd gone through twelve days of pain and had to abandon ship. I waited until my back had recovered and got on rather better with the *Core Abs* DVD that Kiki lent me in which Shiva Rea demonstrated abs of steel on a sun-kissed beach in Kerala as the Indian Ocean lapped her feet. Shiva's third chakra looked pretty good to me and it was clear that deals were landing in her lap, there were several Shiva DVDs on Kiki's shelves and the woman had more signature clothing lines and *Yoga Journal* front covers than any yoga goddess in history.

18

'He lay in bed next to me, chanting the cats' names'

I'd hoped that I would be able to unite the yoga girls of Norfolk and London for the mother of all Hen nights – for when it came down to it those London girls were as much Bad Ladies as the Norfolk girls, but practicalities got in the way so I ended up having two. Normally the chief bridesmaid would be relied upon to organise the Hen but I hadn't appointed one because I couldn't single out any one Bad Lady or Cappuccino Guru; in the end they selected themselves – Poppy volunteered to arrange London and Kiki told me, quite firmly, that she'd be handling the Norwich side of things.

We did Norwich first. The Bad Ladies gathered around a bottle of Prosecco in the bar of Suckling House, a restaurant in the medieval quarter of the city, just round the corner from Baba Ghanoush, the site of my Yogutante party. We stood before the carefully preserved brick, flint and stained-glass windows as Kiki pinned on each of us an official Bad Lady rosette that she'd made – at the centre of which was a photo of me with devilish red horns.

Kate gave me a wooden white hen that I put at the centre of our table in the thirteenth-century courtyard and refused to be parted from all evening. While my outfit involved flared denims, wedges and an off-the-shoulder silk top I'd bought on a trip to Delhi when I was Saving the World from Germs, Kate looked ready for a night on the White Isle, was she heading to Space or Café del Mar after our night out in Norwich? She'd wrapped her slender figure in a slinky white dress that ended in a flamenco-style flare, accessorised with a shell necklace and a white rose tucked behind her ear. She fished around in her beaded bag for some cards – invitations to her forthcoming polytunnel party – featuring a picture of the newly completed hundred-metre-long polytunnel and the suggestion that we bring not a bottle, but a plant. 'It'll be fun,' she enthused, 'I'm cooking, a couple of DJs we met in Ibiza will be playing, there'll be a big dance floor and all our friends and relations will be there.'

We were in.

Kiki had picked up a little gem of a black bustier dress which she'd punked up with a seventies studded belt from her favourite vintage shop, completing the look with large diamante-studded black sunglasses and extreme heels. She looked wonderful, happy in herself, at peace. 'I did the Four Corners Collage,' she explained. 'Kate told me what a difference it made to her, how it helped her to get clear about what she wanted from life and I've done the same. I'm going to cut back my yoga classes – just teach two nights a week, finish up my PhD, and I'm going to get a job as a university lecturer. I want to spend more time satisfying my brain and forget about finding a man – it's such a waste of time, and anyway my son is enough for me. I love spending more time with him, we curl up in our pyjamas with the cats and it's all I need, apart from the odd Tango class.'

Something told me Kiki's man would find her very soon, a handsome university lecturer type in a corduroy jacket, glasses on the end of his nose, a leaking ball-point pen in his pocket. She'd take him to his first-ever Tango class and mid ganchos, barridas and ochos he'd look into her beautiful pale green eyes and find himself in love.

The Angel Wah Wah, an honorary Bad Lady for the night, had no need of further embellishment – she didn't even need a glass of champagne, she was glowing from *nadi* to *nadi*. 'I'm doing the *Kirtin kriya*,' she explained, 'it's the most important meditation in Kundalini yoga – it's designed to remove all traces of past relationships from my subconscious, it restores the arc,' she said, drawing a semi-circle over her head. 'I have to chant "*Sa Ta Na Ma*" thirty-one minutes a day for forty days, ideally for one hundred and twenty, that's how long it takes to transform the body and mind's experience, to integrate it, but I'm fourteen days in and it's already working.' Her husband hadn't taken this restructuring work too seriously; 'He lay in bed next to me, chanting the cats' names in place of "*Sa Ta Na Ma*".'

She pulled a packet of Love tea out of her bag, along with a matching mug that she gave to me with a smile and a hug. What was coming next? I half expected a kettle and hot water but instead she followed up with an announcement. 'Actually, there's another reason I might be glowing,' she added bashfully. 'I'm having a mini-Angel in December.'

The news was met with rapturous applause – especially as it sounded as if the baby might be following in her mother's footsteps; Angel had been for a scan and the nurse had been unable to check the baby's number of fingers as they were held in prayer position.

I checked in with myself – did I need to put on my 'practise and all is coming' T-shirt? No. I felt nothing but delight. 'It seems to be the time for children amongst my friends,' said the Angel Wah Wah, 'apart from one or two who are still prioritising their careers.'

I shook my head, I knew all about that. 'One of them was ninety minutes late for a birthday celebration the other day – she'd been at a work thing and she'd already had three glasses of wine when she arrived – she's thirty and she shows no sign of wanting to settle down. I'm worried about her.'

Me too.

By the end of the meal Kiki, Kate and I had disposed of a couple of bottles of Pinot Grigio and agreed that it would be a good idea to have a post-wedding detox. The Angel Wah Wah suggested a *Pancakarma* retreat in some barns near her house, a plan which was greeted with much enthusiasm – I regretted not having done it earlier in the year and was keen to have some friends with whom I could share the pain. The only sticking point was the length of the retreat. The Angel explained that twenty-eight days was the optimum, but under pressure from us, this was eventually shortened to seven. 'That's the minimum you can do to see any real effect,' advised the Angel.

Deciding that we should continue to abuse our livers until after the wedding we ended the evening in one of Norwich's finest nightclubs. Kate, the only one of us to have tried them all, decided we should do the Ministry of Cheese night at Liquid, one pound to get in before eleven. There had been a few improvements since I last went to a nightclub, in um, 1998, the year that Liquid won UK Nightclub of the Year. The dance floor didn't stick to my feet, the air was no longer thick with cigarette smoke (which gave it the air of a school disco) and the screen beside the dance floor displayed a text number to call – I spent several of my initial dance floor minutes trying to work out why it was there, until Kate used it to text the DJ for some Madonna.

Kate, ever the cool Ibiza chick, alternated between holding a bottle of iced water to her forehead and waving her arms above her head. I tried to copy her perfectly executed moves but couldn't get into the groove as I wasn't able to shake the notion that I was likely to be mistaken for someone's mum – had I got lost on the dance floor coming to pick up one of my children? And then several smartly turned-out lads in their best aftershave clustered around Kate and me, and for a few minutes we were spinning in the vortex of a teenage testosterone fest. It was all very flattering but on balance I was glad I was getting married.

A few days later Poppy, Gabriele, Frances, Andrea and I sat on velvet sofas beneath vast chandeliers in an eighteenth-century salon – a club owned by Poppy's ex-husband and one to which she still belonged. The outfits were as glamorous as the setting – I thought of Kiki and how much she would've loved the show; Poppy in a burnt-orange silk jersey Diane von Furstenberg dress and silver Miu Miu heels, Frances in Louboutins and a chocolate-brown dress with this season's high waisted bow, Andrea in a black silk shift dress with a pretty scoop neck that she'd bought from Edun, a glam eco-chic label, Gabriele in her signature French tailoring, Hermès scarf and loafers, me in jeans, a white leather jacket from Tosho circa 1999, and the Cacharel graphic print top which last summer had prompted the remark, 'I didn't marry Trisha for her tits.'

There was much to celebrate: Andrea's company had launched successfully in Russia, and she'd met an architect who specialised in eco houses at a friend's wedding. There'd been instant chemistry and the all important third date was imminent (cue champagne). Poppy and the Groover from Vancouver were considering a partnership in which they pooled their resources in interior design and architecture to convert a colonial mansion in Kerala into a boutique yoga hotel (cue more champagne). Gabriele was enjoying having more time to herself now that both her children were at school and had been throwing herself into interviewing a range of alpha males – Colin Firth, Leonard Cohen and Charles Saatchi – for her French newspaper. Sadly she refused to give us any non-publishable information but, before she disappeared outside to smoke a cigarette, she did admit that if anything ever happened to her husband Mr Firth might be a contender. Frances had an announcement to make, 'I've got a new album coming out – in fact I wanted to tell you girls about it tonight because it's all rather fitting, actually – it was recorded live at Ronnie Scott's the night that Lucy and David met – I love it – it's all my favourites – a big-band jazz album of old classics.'

Now that was worth another bottle of champagne.

Poppy had booked us a Karma Kar to take us to Momo, the Moroccan institution on Heddon Street. We piled into the back of Tobias's marigold-bedecked, wolf-whistling, burgundy Ambassador and were immediately transported to India – Nag Champa incense blessed our nostrils, evening Ragas blasted our ears, and the Kar's interior burned a psychedelic imprint on our retinas as we bounced around on the red velvet seats, admiring the embroidered door panels and the prints of Bollywood stars smiling dazzlingly from the only surfaces that weren't already covered in gold tassels. Turned out Tobias, a chubby bald man in sunglasses, huge pale pink scarf and white *kurta* pyjamas, had been one of the originals on the hippy trail through India. He'd dreamed up Karma Kars as living proof that the journey was more important than the destination, and by the time we got to Momo, I was in full agreement. I would have been quite happy to have spent the entire Hen night in the back of his car, listening to tales of Goa in the sixties. Actually I would have been happy to have spent the rest of my life in the back of his car – viewed through Tobias's rose-tinted car windows the streets of London were ours for the taking – they were peaceful crime-free places, full of shiny happy people who smiled at us as we passed by; I hadn't felt this excited about the capital since I'd moved here in the mid-eighties. What had happened to the Angry City I left a year ago?

Prising ourselves away from the velvet interiors we were instantly mobbed by more shiny happy people who all wanted to touch the car or have their photo taken beside it. As we made our way into the restaurant I found myself gushing about how much London had changed. 'Now that it's clear I'm not going to be holding children's picnics in fields of poppies anytime soon perhaps I should move back to London, trade my wellies for heels, this season's trowel for a handbag and my Barbour for an oh-so-now coat,' I said, only half joking.

'Don't worry about your clothes, Lucy, you can wear your country wardrobe in town,' observed Poppy. 'Barbours, head-scarves and all things country are always very this season.'

We laughed and sat down to toast the Queen as an enduring icon of country style.

'I don't know,' I said slowly, putting down my glass. 'London is a very different place these days – it seems lighter somehow, more fun, less weighed down by everything.'

'I think you're describing yourself, Lucy,' ventured Frances, smiling. 'Don't you think it might be you that's changed, not London?'

'You seem so much happier, more relaxed, more grounded these days,' added Gabriele, putting her arm round my shoulder.

'It must be all those tree poses you've been doing up in Norfolk,' laughed Andrea.

I agreed. It wasn't just the rose-tinted view through Tobias's windows – something fundamental had shifted inside of me; the thought occurred to me that I could be content wearing both wellies and heels, though perhaps not at the same time. It seemed that London and I had come full circle – now I could see the positives in every negative – I could accept its anonymity in return for its diversity, I could accept the claustrophobia of the Tube in return for emerging onto streets alive with possibilities, I could accept the hard pavements in return for the ability to wear heels unimpeded by mud, I could accept it as a place full of strangers in return for the welcoming embrace of The Cappuccino Gurus, and I could accept it as a place to work long hours in return for knowing I could go home to David.

And what of Norfolk? We had accepted it but had it accepted us? Though the jury was still out it seemed to me that we were on our way – the Sheriff confided in me that he didn't see David as a Paki 'because talking to him you forget his skin colour; perhaps it's the tweed cap he wears but I think of him as one of us.' Whether we'd been absorbed by

Norfolk or not I knew that Norfolk was now in every bone of my body, bar perhaps my hands which continued to feel more comfortable holding a handbag than a garden trowel.

I realised that I didn't want to choose between Norfolk and London, and actually, I didn't have to. Perhaps it was time to bring together The Bad Ladies and The Cappuccino Gurus into one super group – reflecting the best of both places, the best of each other and the best of me. I would provisionally title it the *Handbag and Wellies Yoga Club*, pending their approval. I thought they'd be happy with it – after all The Bad Ladies did handbags with enviable flare – Kiki had a collection to rival any film-noir heroine and Kate's were the tiniest – and nearly always on a cord worn sideways across her body so that she could wave both hands in the air at any given moment. Meanwhile The Cappuccino Gurus all did a nice line in Wellington boots – Poppy had the silver pair that she'd worn with her pink kaftan for a walk around our woods, Gabriele's were Le Chameau 'naturellement', and Andrea hadn't yet found a fair-trade organic pair but contented herself with the fact they were green, at least.

Returning to Norfolk the following night I sat in the garden contemplating the full moon casting a silvery light over the rose bushes. Clasping my mug of peppermint tea against the chill in the air I remembered an old saying – that the people we surround ourselves with tell us who we are. I thought about The Bad Ladies of Norfolk and The Cappuccino Gurus and it struck me that none of us were like-minded about everything or even the same in very many ways – and yet, despite our different relationships with men and the wide range of life choices we'd made, it seemed clear to me that we were all on the same path, all trying to be the best people we could be, and with that intention the distances that can lie between human beings had been reduced to the breadth of a yoga mat.

We'd shared our ups and our downs, sometimes with more complexity than was strictly necessary, and always with more Pinot Grigio than was strictly necessary. Although we weren't always at peace with ourselves we were working our way towards it and supporting each other along the way. We'd all made difficult choices in our lives, and some of us had been guilty of making non-choices. None of us had got everything we wanted in life, but we celebrated what we had, individually and collectively. Yes, everyone seemed to be moving on to a new and significant stage in their lives but there was no point in wishing it any other way – our friendship lay not in the desire for each other's company or in the fear of losing it but in acceptance, whatever the circumstance.

My own development had been no exception. As I looked back over the year that had been it was clear to me that experience had been a great teacher; I'd created a new inner life – not the one that I'd originally intended, the little bundle of joy for whom I was going to hold idyllic parties in fields of poppies, but nonetheless a new way of seeing that had transformed me, allowing me to accept myself as I am – a forty-something woman who'd met her love too late to have children of her own but who aspired to be a universal mother to all children, a woman who was already a fully paid-up member of Chaka Khan's 'I'm Every Woman' sisterhood, a woman who individually was something, who collectively was everything, a woman with every freedom available to her, a woman blessed to be able to exercise choice in being the person she wanted to be.

19

'I will'

Somehow, despite the fact that we were planning a home-spun affair involving just fifty adults and a few children, the week before the wedding was fraught and frantic. I spent several nights lying awake worrying whether I'd told every-one that the service started at 2.30... if the directions to the church were clear... where I should seat my many rela-tives, my parents, brothers, half-brothers, stepsisters and David's family. When I wasn't worrying about everyone else, I was worrying about myself – fixating on the moment I would walk down the aisle with all eyes upon me. I became obsessed with my appearance. Would my arms be buff enough? How many applications of fake tan would I need? When should I start the applications? Should I wear my hair up or down? Would my dress fit me? I'd never been so vain.

I lost about half a stone as time set aside for eating became a luxury I felt I could do without. David managed to eat but was clearly feeling the strain. He developed dark shadows under his eyes as he fought to combine his business's busiest time of the year with calls to the marquee guy, the barbecue guy, the cable guy... We began to row over the smallest details and, while we didn't question the wisdom of getting married (well, only for an hour at a time), we wondered more than once why we hadn't taken the easy option and held the reception in a venue built for the purpose?

I was filled with new-found admiration for the people behind marquee events – who but the English could dream up such an eccentric idea? I wondered how the first people to decide to have a marquee wedding reception had got there...

'Where shall we hold the reception? In our house, or perhaps at the local restaurant, or maybe in the ballroom at the local hotel?'

'Oooh – that would be far too easy. I know, let's build a restaurant from nothing in the middle of a field, ideally located miles from electricity or water supplies, and let's put in chandeliers, a dance floor and a bar.'

I veered from abject panic to wide-eyed fascination and back again as said restaurant, bar and dance floor were constructed from scratch on our lawn. A team of four extra-strong men arrived and erected the marquee in a day – the hottest day of the year – consuming endless cups of piping hot and sugared tea as the temperature soared into the thirties, standing on ladders to hang the chandeliers and decorate the canvas with swags of cream chiffon, crawling on their hands and knees to lay a vast thirty-six by thirty-two-foot dance floor the even surface of which would, we hoped, preserve the safety of the high-heeled and the old.

An endless stream of specialists arrived and did their thing – forty crates containing precise amounts of rented crockery and cutlery were piled high atop circular tables and gilt-backed chairs. A Land Rover deposited a walk-in refrigerated trailer at the back of the marquee along with two vast state-of-the-art barbecues, two tubby men carefully wheeled their disco and light set across the uneven grass, the generator arrived – the subject of some debate. I'd had visions of the entire marquee plunging into darkness as it failed to cope with the demands of the disco lights, chandeliers and water boilers and considered spending £500 on a forty-five KVA generator, which our marquee guy recommended. Once David had established that the wedding business thrives on two things – fear and ignorance – fear that something might go wrong on the 'special day' and ignorance on the part of the bride and groom in not knowing their arse from their KVA, it was clear that a six KVA would do just fine. Once it was all up and running I wished we'd thought of putting it to more use – my mother could've filmed another one of her Hollywood blockbusters here – there was enough room in the refrigerated trailer for a thousand pink sticky buns and at least one handsome French chef.

Work outside the marquee was just as epic in scale; the garden still needed some work and although David loved strimming the edges of the grass in his orange hard hat and goggles bought specially for the purpose, he didn't have time to do everything that needed doing. The grass had been long engaged in a summer growth spurt, some beds needed planting and the rabbit-proof fence needed mending – the lawn often resembled a scene from *Watership Down*, except our rabbit community didn't seem to be suffering any shortage of does. We needed a strong man to come and help. I asked the Sheriff for a recommendation and the very next day, at seven in the morning, a large pick-up truck roared up the drive. A six-foot-something shaven-headed man emerged. He walked towards me with an alarming lilt to the left, the man had clearly only got one leg. He got closer – he had an eyebrow piercing, a tattoo of a red-eyed devil smoking a cigar on the side of his neck, three gold knuckle dusters on the fingers of his left hand, and his right hand had been replaced by a silver hook. Should I run? I found myself rooted to the spot. He smiled, his gold-capped teeth glinting in the morning sun. 'I'm Jimmy,' he said, holding out his left hand, 'the Sheriff told me you need some help in the garden?'

Jimmy the One-Armed Gardener worked solidly until 5.30, accomplishing more in ten hours than a man with all his limbs gets done in a week. By the end of the week, accompanied by a small team of lads, he'd mended all the fences, planted the beds and covered the drive in twenty-six tonnes of gravel – I couldn't understand why it was taking so long until I realised he was using a rake to spread it. I concluded that Jimmy was in training to become a Buddhist monk and had begun practising Zen and the Art of Pea Shingle Maintenance.

I painted the garden gate wearing a straw cowboy hat, bikini top and shorts, still trying to lose some unsightly strap marks before W Day – Zara Philips had attempted to set a new trend in this area at her brother's wedding but it had left me cold. I was rather proud of my look until the Sheriff called by and deemed me 'a hillbilly'. It could've been worse; a sweaty David, shovelling pea shingle while sporting a thick beard, a pair of shorts rolled up like a loin cloth and a T-shirt wrapped around his head, was universally agreed to look like Norfolk's first-ever *dalit* – a member of the Untouchable caste.

The Sheriff beamed from ear to ear.

'You look happy,' said David.

'I've just been to see my babies,' he explained. 'I have 5,200 of them.'

We agreed that this was an impressive number, especially for a man of the Sheriff's age.

'So what stage are your babies at?' I asked.

'They're poults,' he said helpfully.

'Poults?'

'Poults are bigger than chicks, they have their feathers and can fly,' he explained, patiently.

'So what happens to them now?' I asked.

'They are in pens getting acclimatised. Then when they are ten weeks old we will move them out into the fields in small batches, taking care where we put them – we don't want them wandering onto the road.'

'Then what happens?' I asked.

'Then,' he smiled broadly, his face turning pink with pleasure, 'the shooting season begins.'

The Sheriff was a brave man – there was no way I could nurture 5,200 little birds knowing most of them would be shot in a matter of weeks.

'You don't fancy doing a bit of beating next season do you?' he asked.

I replied that I didn't. The idea of watching those beautiful birds falling out of the sky appalled me.

He tried again. 'The trailer is going to be very high-tech this year – it will have individual seats with a bar, a gun rack and two dog kennels at the front. Perhaps you could drive it for us?'

It was a skill I had yet to pick up.

'How about helping the man who runs the game cart?

He's not good on his pins these days; he needs an assistant to pick up the dead birds.'

I thanked him for the opportunity and informed him that, regretfully, his suggestion had done nothing to change my mind.

Sensing he was getting nowhere he changed tack. 'You haven't got a French maid's outfit have you? You could wear it to serve up lunch to the beaters – it might give the old boys the energy to get through the rest of the afternoon.'

Sadly I didn't.

I managed to squeeze in a couple of yoga classes the week before the wedding. Kiki's Tuesday night class was packed, full of people and Kiki-isms:

'Good breath-work class – you sound as if you are one person, which of course you are, yogically speaking.'

'Do a half vinyasa – it's like the sorbet between courses.'

'A smile will lift your legs another inch.'

We performed *Kurmasana*, or Tortoise Pose, sliding our shoulders beneath our knees and resting our faces on the floor, actually I watched as the rest of the class slid their shoulders beneath their knees and rested their faces on the floor, and then we all watched as the only man in the room popped his ankles behind his ears and lifted himself up so that he could swing back and forwards. We laughed and sighed, and reminded ourselves of the old adage: 'practise and all is coming.' Kiki's own practice was seemingly effortless, she'd jump from *Bhujapidasana* to *Chaturanga Dandasana* in one easy flowing move as the rest of us looked on enviously. I thought she looked awesome but she was convinced that she'd put on half a stone and planned another one-month detox after the wedding – not the Angel Wah Wah's *Pancakarma* but Carol Vorderman's *Detox For Life*.

Three days before the wedding I went to Kate's last-ever class at the Quaker Meeting House. By her own admission she was now 'very much the country girl' but, from the moment she bowed her head and said '*Namaste*' I was headed straight to the Bermuda Triangle, via Ibiza. The one thing I definitely recall was managing three sets of three full press-ups – it may not sound like much but for me it was a triumph, and a testimony to Kiki's buff arms programme, at least that was one less thing to worry about. We ended with a long meditation – while once I ran scream-ing for the hills I was now able to sit still and listen to the sound of my breath; it was still a little uneven but there had definitely been an improvement. When the others had left we two Bad Ladies drew together and hugged. I had expected tears, certainly on my part, but there were none – we were moving on with our lives and everything was as it was meant to be.

Walking back to my car accompanied by the peal of St Michael's church bells, I did feel a certain sadness, an era had come to an end; the middle of my week would have a big hole in it now and I would miss the other girls in the class – I was sorry that I would only get to read about our baker's prizes in the local press and that I would probably never hear whether the two sixteen-year-olds passed all their exams with flying colours, though something told me they would. I comforted myself with the thought that I had a friend for life in Kate and that she already seemed so settled in her new home, complete with polytunnel.

*

I'd decided to follow with tradition and spend the night before the wedding away from home – in Dad and Nikki's attic suite at Fritton House, the local boutique hotel. My bedroom was a lovely room built into the eaves of the house with views out over fields and sheep, no matter that it lacked essential amenities like wardrobes and coat hangers. I felt guilty indulging in such tranquillity when there was plenty still to be done at home. I told myself that David may have been left with a morning's work ahead of him but I'd done a lot when he was still in London. Besides, I'd left him a list of what needed to be done and, I reasoned, he could ask his brothers, who were staying at the house, for help. What could possibly go wrong?

I woke up on Saturday morning feeling well rested and excited but nervous. Would all the guests find the church? Would I be able to walk up the aisle in my Jimmy Choos? Would I fluff my vows? Would my fake tan have left orange marks on the back of my ankles? Would David manage to get to the church before me? I took some deep breaths, contemplated doing some yoga, thought better of it, ordered some tea from room service, tried not to listen to my father rehearsing his speech in the next room, and settled back down in bed to read the wedding service for the fiftieth time. I was half way through the sixty-sixth psalm when the phone calls from a careworn and hung-over-sounding David began.

'Babe – no need to panic but the new shower has flooded the hall…'

'Babe – how do I get constant hot water?'

'Babe – where's the Order of Service? No one can find it.'

It was time to get up.

*

I looked out of the breakfast room window – the sheep were huddled together and dark grey clouds threatened the horizon. What had happened to the previous fortnight's clear blue skies and record-breaking temperatures?

'Not to worry, Lucy,' said Dad brightly, putting down his paper momentarily to butter some toast, 'the rain will be done by lunchtime.'

I was too nervous to eat but three cups of tea and a cappuccino got me going and while Nikki finished her breakfast and my father the scientist sat in his bedroom with Quynh, the Vietnamese photographer introduced to us by Kiki, discussing Metaheuristics in Feature Construction and Clustering (the subject of Quynh's PhD) I had a shower and a blow dry.

Kate had sent me her hairdresser, the woman responsible for her trademark long blonde waves. After much consultation and several trial runs in which I'd attempted the hair of a Grecian goddess, a chignon-toting glamour queen from the 1940s and a ringleted romantic, I'd finally decided to go as myself and wear it down. 'You want to be the best of you, not a different person,' advised Kate's Mistress of the Waves wisely. She was also a mistress of the volume-boosting blow dry and managed to transform my head of fine straight hair into something approaching an abundance of luxurious thick waves. Nikki also had need of her skills when her plan to wear a feather fascinator went awry – she walked into the huge bathroom in which I'd set up camp and we both fell about laughing – it was fascinating for all the wrong reasons – as if a bird had nested in her hair – not a great look, especially for one of the mothers of the bride.

I'd decided to do my own make-up following a couple

of unsuccessful trial runs with local make-up artists in which I'd ended up looking rather unlike myself. I had to take it very slowly on account of my shaking hands, but in the end I managed a passable imitation of a Lancôme look – all smoky eyes and pale lips – that I'd seen in last week's *Grazia*. I hadn't meant to buy an entirely new set of brushes as well as an entirely new make-up collection but the lovely lady in John Lewis had been so helpful... and there'd been an offer on... and well, it *was* my wedding day...

Make-up and hair done but still in my dressing gown I had half an hour to spare and so my brother, his wife Jo, Millie and Teddy popped up to see us. Teddy brought a juice he'd personally ordered at the bar, and while he sat sweetly on the miniature sofa keeping an eye on his sleeping little sister, we adults stood beneath the eaves attempting to stand up straight and drink a glass of champagne. I seemed to get more of it on my dressing gown than in my mouth owing to nerves and eventually gave up.

It was time to put on my dress. I looked in the mirror and once again thanked Kiki for the buff-arms programme and its delightful boob lifting and expanding side effects. My bouquet of blush roses, freesia and hypericum berries arrived, held together by a cream ribbon and tiny pins and, as Nikki got dressed, Dad played mind-training games and Quynh took portrait shots of my Jimmy Choos and the fabulous gold necklace the Hugging Mother had lent me, I sat barefoot in my bedroom admiring my pedicured feet and gathering my thoughts. I was still nervous, too nervous to be able to eat the sandwich that Nikki ordered for me, but I was beginning to feel a little calmer – there were heart-warming texts from the Angel Wah Wah and Gabriele on their respective

Mediterranean beaches. I was sorry not to be sharing the day with them, especially with Gabriele, whose own wedding in the City of Light, gorging on sugared almond favours called dragées and a traditional French wedding cake of profiteroles and caramel, had been so magical. There'd been no further calls from David so I assumed that everything at the house was under control, and as I settled, I began to look forward to seeing everyone, especially my mum who'd driven down from north Norfolk that morning and was with Jessica, now nearly one, and my very pregnant stepsister at the B&B round the corner from our house.

I left the sandwich and almost full glass of champagne (something of a first in my family) and said 'goodbye and thank you for finding me a clothes rail and some hangers' to the staff at the hotel. Dad handed me into the vintage Rolls Royce which was now glistening in the weak sun. The car belonged to Lol, a family friend who enjoyed putting his most prized possession to good use. I placed my Lancôme shopping bag, full of eyeshadow, waterproof mascara and Polo mints, at my feet. The three suitcases and yoga mat that I'd evidently felt I needed for the overnight stay went in the boot and off we went. I thought there might follow some last-minute fatherly advice but Dad talked Rolls Royce engineering with Lol – I expect he thought that he'd given enough advice to me over the past forty-odd years, and I'd have to agree with him. Instead he took my hand and held it all the way to the church, another first, and I was nothing but grateful; I couldn't actually have conducted a conversation as my mouth was so dry.

Despite a detour to the McDonald's roundabout for a bottle of water I still managed to arrive at the church a minute early, getting there before Andrea and Frances, who'd got lost on the way up to Norfolk, then gone to the other Catholic church – the one in the centre of Beccles – leaving them with no time and no choice but to get changed in McDonald's. They came running up the hill in their heels and hats, the Dom looked on in his golden cloak – more golden than my dress – hinting at disbelief with a smiling shake of the head. I could tell that he recognised a couple of Bad Ladies when he saw them.

I peered inside the church – it looked like a florist's; our friend Joanna had given us five hundred Avalanche roses in white and blush pink as a wedding present. Mrs Organ and her team had arranged them, along with oriental lilies, freesia, lysianthus and hypericum berries, into urns, onto pedestals, along the altar rails, and made them up as huge hearts that now decorated the nineteenth-century wrought-iron balustrades. It looked beautiful and I would like to say serene, but I'd be lying – the place was chaos. The Order of Service scrolls that the Hugging Mother had spent half a day rolling and wrapping in golden ribbon, had got lost en route to the church. Finally they'd arrived and now both scrolls and the ushers responsible for them were bundling down the aisles with unseemly haste. I felt a surge of panic and had to fight a sudden urge to run into the church and give them a hand but Dad and the Dom restrained me. 'Leave them to it – they'll sort it out,' said the Dom, smiling in the manner of one who'd seen it all before.

Finally everyone had their Order of Service, the crowd settled and the Dom, Dad and I moved to the church door. I saw David waiting at the altar rails, he turned to me and smiled and I knew, in that moment, that it was all going to be all right – that the service would be all right, that the reception would be all right and that the rest of my life would most definitely be all right. He looked so handsome in his blue shirt and lightweight brown corduroy suit, bought in Palma's Massimo Dutti on a summer holiday last year, he looked emotional – his chest high, his big brown eyes welling up, he looked happy to be surrounded by family and friends, he looked happy to see me – if only because he'd never have to worry about mislaying important pieces of paper again.

The musicians struck up Richard Wagner's 'Lohengrin', otherwise known as 'Here Comes the Bride', the Dom began his slow walk towards the altar and I was ready to walk down the aisle. The music spilled out of church, almost visible in the sudden burst of sunshine, encircling Dad and me and transporting us towards David on a wave of heavenly notes. I caught my breath at the sight of so many Bad Ladies, Cappuccino Gurus, family and friends gathered together in the tiny church – I tried to smile at everyone individually but had to give up because there were loved ones at every turn. All I could take in was a sea of smiles and the vivid colours lit up by camera flashes; Poppy's fuchsia and orange Diane von Furstenberg, Kiki in a green silk vintage slip dress and, judging by her height, killer heels, the Divine Child by her side sporting a pink jumper and blue checked golfing trousers, Kate in a slinky floor-length white number, Andrea in a pewter silk wrapover dress, Frances in a floral maxi dress and huge felt hat, the Hugging Mother in an olive-green and pink sari, Nikki in cool grey lace and pearls, and there was my mother, every inch the leading lady, channelling Dior's New Look in a cobalt-blue silk dress.

I arrived by David's side and suddenly the rest of the

church fell away. It was just me and him, just him and me, just the two of us, side by side.

Quynh managed to move around the church taking pictures without disturbing anyone (thank goodness he'd changed out of the canary yellow Norwich Football Club shirt he'd worn to the rehearsal) but one of David's oldest friends decided to make an unscheduled appearance at the altar and film the entire service from the Dom's side. The Dom exhibited great forbearance, exchanging 'I'm pained but trying not to take this intrusion into God's house too seriously' looks with us. Our soloist sang the psalm 'Let all the Peoples Praise You' and we all joined in for the hymns – my favourite 'Praise my Soul the King of Heaven' and David's favourite 'Lord of all Hopefulness, Lord of all Joy'. Hearing everyone we knew singing their hearts out on our behalf made my voice wobble and my eyes fill up and I had to press my buff arm against David's lightweight corduroy sleeve to steady myself.

The Dom began his address with references to the book of Genesis, in which 'God created order out of chaos' and admitted to an initial concern that 'chaos would win the day when the Order of Service appeared eternally lost'. He also admitted to feeling 'slightly nervous' because one of his 'greatest critics was about to get married. After every Sunday mass, *if* he's arrived on time, he enjoys enormously telling me the theological heresies that I have given in my sermon.' He didn't seem unduly worried by David's potential criticisms of this address, advising him to 'wait until the last judgement to know if he's correct or not'. He was kinder to me; referring to 'the remarkable self-discipline of yoga' and admitting that this was 'something you can see by my figure

I don't have in anyway whatsoever'. The address was universally declared to contain the best words on marriage that anyone had ever heard and was so compelling that an Afghani princess, who'd recently been married in a Muslim ceremony, said she'd have liked a church wedding herself. I was sure that the Dom would've obliged – he'd readily agreed with David's suggestion that we hear Jewish and Muslim Bidding Prayers at the end of the service.

My six-year-old nephew Teddy bore the rings, wearing a striped shirt and waistcoat, but seemed rather more interested in the Dom's golden cloak than in the details of the wedding ceremony. David said 'I do' and I said 'I will', we struggled with sliding the rings on to each other's fingers – is there something about nerves that makes them expand? We both wiped away some tears, and 'I now pronounce you man and wife' was greeted with a jump for joy from me, a hug from David and a long round of applause and cheers from the congregation. Eventually the Dom broke up the hug and we led the exodus from the church as if we were lit from within by a million diamonds.

I donned David's tweed cap as protection against the sudden shower of confetti which arrived in another burst of sunshine and Teddy leapt into our arms. I wouldn't have cared if it had tipped with rain – I was over the moon, the stars, and the sun. During the photo call the church bells pealed, which initially confused me as the church doesn't have bells; finally I worked out that they were coming from Lol's Rolls Royce – he had a tape machine in the car. There was keen competition for my bouquet but in the end Andrea triumphed, leaping into the air with a velocity that defied Kiki and gravity. Eventually we ran out of people to hug and

Teddy, who'd spent most of his time being the centre of attention, decided he'd rather ride with us than go in his father's BMW, perhaps more to do with the Rolls Royce than us.

I'd only been away a night but I was so glad to return to the farmhouse, to feel the heavy crunch of gravel beneath the Rolls, to see the garden waiting quietly for its big moment, to be carried over the threshold and to have a couple of minutes alone with David. We stood at our bedroom window looking out at the willow tree in front of the house as Billa purred and drooled, walking slow figures of eight around my ankles. We watched the waitresses dashing back and forth to the marquee with trays of food and buckets of ice, perhaps unnecessary given the chill in the air. We looked at each other, squeezed hands and knew that we were, in every sense of the word, home.

Our sense of secure serenity was short-lived. Chaos followed us around that day like a small but persistent Terrier. The neighbouring farm's estate manager had kindly arranged to let us use the area in front of the farm's storage barns as a car park and had even suspended a grain delivery so that our access wouldn't be disturbed. Sadly, the ushers hadn't been briefed to send traffic that way so cars were beginning to cluster on the farmhouse drive, a situation that soon created a tailback worthy of the M25 on a rainy Friday night. The Dom stepped into the breach – directing all the cars back up the track wearing his now plain black cloth and exhibiting an efficiency that came from years of herding unruly flocks.

Once guests had managed to navigate their way out of the car park they found themselves in the midst of a very English wedding. The weather held while we drank champagne on the lawn, though my Jimmy Choos kept sinking dangerously into the mud. It held again until Dad's speech, when torrential rain poured down on the marquee. Perhaps it was divine intervention to keep everyone inside until he'd finished as he outlined every single key moment in my history, beginning with the name my mother gave me when she was pregnant ('Buddleia'), outlining the early years in which I frequently crawled beneath my cot to sleep, 'perhaps an early indication of a yearning for the hard floor of a yoga studio', and ending with my continuing ability to persuade him to buy me a glossy magazine whenever we pass a newsagent together.

Kiki made a speech about how she thought I was the woman who ran off with her boyfriend in Mysore and forgot to say that I *wasn't* the woman who ran off with her boyfriend in Mysore. Poppy read a Rumi poem about planting trees and brought in a bunch of helium-filled heart-shaped red balloons that we released with the help of Teddy and the Divine Child. My stepfather Oliver read out a poem by Indian poet Rabindranath Tagore and spoke of being amused to see a headline in *The Times* recently, 'Mascarenhas puts Edge in the driving seat', which he'd brought with him for all to see... 'David, you have been warned.' David hadn't had any time to prepare a speech so he spoke from the heart, thankfully avoiding all references to his Indian accountant's comment that he was 'marrying a spinster', calling me his 'beautiful wife' and bringing tears to my eyes, again.

I broke with tradition and made a short speech, describing the emotions that came with changing my name. I talked about the honour I felt in having been an Edge – about the high standards set by my parents – the value my father placed on education and how he'd one day let go of the reins, giving me the freedom to explore, but always been by my side even when I was on the other side of the world, and how he taught me the importance of holding out for what I wanted – even if it took more than forty years to find it. I talked about my mum, who'd been an Edge for fourteen years, how she had many talents, and how many of them had eluded me; that while I can't so much as walk onstage without getting stage fright she'd just concluded a ten-day stint at the Maddermarket Theatre getting rave reviews for her role as Mrs Fitzpatrick in *Tom Jones*, that while I am tone deaf she can sing, that while I can't thread a needle she can turn her hand to making just about anything from costumes to curtains, and that she has a special talent for finding great men – first my father, and then Oliver – my other father, chief inspector of treacle tarts, student of Anglo-Saxon, speaker of Russian and occasional pantomime dame. I talked about my other mother Nikki, whose wide-ranging talents took her from her own prestigious PR company in London to the Harlow Magistrates Court (where, I hastened to add, she was on the bench not in front of it). I talked about her desire to create better relationships, to make the world a better place, and the fact that she had never been short of a word on any subject – skills that found an outlet at the Stepfamilies Association, a hospice and with me. It may have taken her thirty years but she'd played a significant part in getting me to the point I could say 'I will' to the man I love.

Then I talked about the honour in being a Mascarenhas; about David's father breaking the story of the genocide in East Pakistan – a story splashed across the front page of the

Sunday Times – at great risk to himself and his family. I told everyone that I wished that I had known him but in the end it was consolation enough to love the people who loved, and continue to love him. I talked about his wife Yvonne, my Hugging Mother, being called upon to leave behind everything she'd ever known and carry five children and two suitcases from Karachi to Ladbroke Grove, and how, despite all of this she remained the happiest person I know; whether she was joyriding the London buses, filling me with tea and Cynthia's samosas or gliding around John Lewis, she was always radiant, always full of grace, and always stunningly beautiful, without so much as a wrinkle at seventy-seven. And then I talked about my love for David, the man I fell for in the queue outside Ronnie Scott's, 'The man who picks me up when I am down, or in John Lewis, the man who, should I ever be in any doubt, has a point of view on all of life's dilemmas, the man who is so deeply a part of me that I no longer feel entirely myself without him.'

After a wedding breakfast of local beef, chicken and lamb barbecued with military precision by our chef Robert Oberhoffer (an army man turned restaurateur whose time served in the Gulf War stood him in good stead for any eventuality), the gilt chairs and white linen tables were pushed to the sides, the candles and lanterns were lit, and David and I took to the floor for our slow dance. For a time we'd nursed ambitions of putting on a *Strictly Come Dancing* style performance, ambitions that we were stripped of when we took our first dance lesson and found me to be strictly rubbish at learning even the most basic choreography. We were tempted to ask everyone to join us for some straightforward *Strictly Strumpy*-style line dancing but worried that our guests would be unable to curb their enthusiasm sufficiently. So we hugged each other close as we danced to Fleetwood Mac's 'Landslide' and David kept pinching my bum – not a move that would've been popular with the *Strictly* judges but the crowd loved it and thank goodness they took quickly en masse to the extensive dance floor, amply fuelled by our friend Kevin's wedding present to us – a hundred bottles of wine and thirty bottles of champagne, and by Cynthia's triumph of a cake, which featured three tiers of chocolate traced with Kashmiri lace icing, resulting in a fight (not just amongst the children) for the first slice.

The yoga girls were united on the dance floor – led by Kate during the Ibiza anthems set, by Frances during the Bee Gees medley and by Kiki, who led Andrea in an all too brief Tango demonstration. 'Dancing Queen' had my mother and I channelling Agnetha and Frida, Oliver and Nikki gave Sonny and Cher's 'I've Got You, Babe' their own magic, Shania Twain's 'You're Still The One' had the Groover from Vancouver leading Poppy in a perfectly executed Canadian Smooth, and Kate and Will glided around the dance floor to the strains of Wet Wet Wet's 'Love is All Around'. Each of us was at home in our chosen decade, apart from Dad who turned out to have mastered all the decades. He displayed a startling amount of energy for a man in his seventies – jiving simultaneously with Nikki, Cynthia and the Hugging Mother, surrounding himself with Bad Ladies, attempting to throw me across his back and over his shoulder in a dance manoeuvre last seen in *Grease*. I had *no* idea he was such a sharp mover.

Teddy and the Divine Child manned the bar pouring drinks for the swelling numbers of Bad Ladies in a manner that led me to question whether their parents had adopted the same approach to education as my father. As a man with several honorary degrees, he'd started my education young, teaching me to read when I was two – largely, I suspect, so that I would be able to assemble his drinks correctly. He used handwritten show cards such as these:

Gin
Tonic (just a splash)
Rioja
Claret
Burgundy
Dom Perignon
Sauvignon Blanc

Seeing so many parents with their children gave me a few pangs but I mentally put on my 'practise and all is coming' T-shirt, stood quietly alone for a few minutes, watching Teddy and the Divine Child taking a break from their bar duties for a game of football, and the pangs drifted away.

The small dog called Chaos stayed away until late in the evening – when the waitresses decided to go home without serving the evening buffet, leaving David and I to serve up hundreds of lamb koftas, when the taxi company we'd booked for the duration refused to return from a far-flung job, leaving guests stranded for several hours, and when I discovered that the huge pile of hand towels I had put aside for the loos had remained in storage and guests had used the same one over and over for ten hours.

On the upside no one seemed in the least bit bothered. David's friend Handsome Harry propositioned Frances and

Andrea – offering them a once-in-a-lifetime opportunity to take part in a threesome, which they chose to decline. The disco went on until two in the morning, the Afghani princess, her husband and Frances leading a Tequila drinking competition resulting in a series of photos that looked more like a night at Space than an English country wedding. Those suffering from sore feet found relief in the warmth of the kitchen where my father opened more bottles, Cynthia and Nikki handed round wedding cake and hot pastries to the needy and Billa leapt from lap to lap. David and I would've loved to stay up all night but eventually complete exhaustion overtook us and we retired to bed with the party still in full swing. Lying in each other's arms we replayed the highlights of the day and, despite the enthusiastic presence of Chaos the Terrier, we concluded that it was quite the best wedding either of us had ever had.

Even with the untiring help of Cynthia and the Hugging Mother it took us two days to clean the marquee, find all the now rotten boxes of food the waitresses had failed to put out for the buffet and count all the teaspoons and corks (we'd drunk ninety bottles of Kevin's wine and all thirty bottles of champagne – not bad for fifty adults).

Finally, David had to go back to London and work on the Wednesday. I watched him leave, and in an attempt to stem the sobs that threatened to carry his car all the way back to London, I made myself a trusty mug of peppermint tea and sat for a while. As I contemplated the insect life fluttering around the newly imported water lilies in our little pond I thought about each of my spiritual epiphanies – I'd learned the art of acceptance, I'd tasted the cosmic bliss of universal motherhood, and I knew that I could channel Chaka Khan's 'I'm Every Woman' whenever I was having an envious moment. I wondered, given the considerable spiritual progress I'd made, whether Norfolk was the new India – I could see the advertising slogan now:

'Experience the true wisdom of the East – come to Norfolk.'

There was no need to don a dirty dhoti, join Osho's Brotherhood of the White Robes or squat on a sacred *ghat*, in this county enlightenment would find you. You might be on a pink mat in The Lotus Room, you might be following the yellow socks on a cold November day, you might be in a white leather-clad karaoke bar – wherever you found yourself there was sure to be a ready supply of spiritual juice, as delicious as Norfolk cider.

Perhaps Tobias could come and have a spiritual epiphany here too; he'd remodel his Karma Kars; paint them all green and bedeck them with garlands of plastic poppies. Inside there'd be glorious Technicolor pictures of holy Simmental cows, there'd be big blue skies on the ceiling and grass on the seats, there'd be the musky smell of rapeseed in the incense burner and on the dashboard there'd be pictures of the county's spiritual shrines – The Lotus Room, Somerleyton Hall, and Sing Sing karaoke bar – and its gurus – the Sheriff, the Dom and The Bad Ladies. Tobias would spread the word amongst his celebrity clients; Kate Moss, John McEnroe and Ronaldo; they'd make their way up the slow road to nowhere and they too would learn the art of acceptance as they sat behind a tractor doing ten miles an hour.

As I watched the sun casting long shadows over the lawn it seemed to me that while I might have lost the egg and womb race I was still a winner. I'd moved from a tiny flat to a beautiful farmhouse, I'd made the transition from single girl to married woman, I'd gained some newly buff arms, but the best win had been much bigger than that. Okay, so there wasn't going to be a baby for David and me, but I'd discovered a new-found appreciation for everything that I have and, instead of chasing after what wasn't possible I'd accepted what was, and counted myself very lucky. I had a husband who loved me as I am, without expectation and without false hope. I had better relationships with my old friends and family, I had growing relationships with new friends and a new family and, at last, I had my very own Hugging Mother, without the need to queue. I'd worked out what was truly important in my life, and though I still didn't feel as comfortable with a trowel as I did with a hand-bag I was as comfortable in wellies as I'd been in heels, though perhaps I'd always feel most comfortable with bare feet on my yoga mat, surrounded by Bad Ladies and Cappuccino Gurus, with David in my heart.

The Hugging Mother's Recipe for Mangalorean Prawn Curry

This recipe has been adapted by my mother Yvonne from my great-grandmother's famous prawn curry. Evelyn Domingo was very particular about ingredients, using fresh coconut in her curries which she ground on a stone along with the other spices.

She liked Kashmiri red chillies for their flavour – they're milder than most chillies and give curries a wonderful red colour which, when combined with turmeric, looks like a setting sun. Kashmiri chillies can be substituted with red chilli powder and sweet paprika, but it's always worth a journey to Southall for the real thing.

My mother has given my great-grandmother's recipe the urban housewife's touch, substituting grated coconut for coconut milk or cream. Watching her make it on special occasions taught me that cooking is truly a labour of love. I hope that you enjoy it too, and continue our tradition.

Cynthia Mascarenhas

Serves six

Ingredients
1 medium onion finely sliced
5 or 6 fresh curry leaves

4 large plum tomatoes – chopped
2 tablespoons tomato puree (the bottles are better than the little tins and tubes)
1 teaspoon sugar
1 medium can unsweetened coconut milk
½ kg peeled raw King Prawns, heads off

For the seasoning:
A few drops of fish sauce
Lime juice if preferred
Fresh coriander roughly chopped

Vegetable oil for the pan

For the red masala paste (if you are in a hurry 30g of Patak's Kashmiri masala curry paste with chilli and garlic is a useful substitute)

5 or 6 red Kashmiri chillies, seeds removed **or** 4 tablespoons of red chilli powder and 1 tablespoon sweet paprika
5 cloves garlic
½ inch fresh ginger
4 or 5 peppercorns
2 medium onions sliced (plus the onion set aside for frying)
1½ tablespoons ground coriander powder
1 teaspoon ground cumin
2 teaspoons turmeric
2 tablespoons white wine vinegar
1 teaspoon tamarind – deseeded

Combine all of the masala ingredients in a food processor and grind until smooth. It is important that the chillies, ginger and garlic be as pulverised as possible with no little bits. Add the white wine vinegar and blend again until very smooth. Transfer to a bowl.

Heat the vegetable oil in a large heavy-based saucepan until hot but not smoking. Sprinkle over the curry leaves; allow them to splutter for a few seconds. Add 1 finely sliced onion, fry until soft and golden. Add the red masala paste, give it a good stir and cook for 15 minutes over a medium to low heat. The idea is that the spices cook gently and slowly release their oils.

Now turn up the heat to medium, stir in the chopped tomatoes, sugar and tomato puree. Continue cooking for 5 minutes until they have softened and blended with the masala.

Add the coconut milk to the pan. Let it simmer gently for about 20 minutes until the curry is slowly thickened.

Add the raw prawns and continue to simmer for 10 minutes. Or if you prefer to cook the prawns first just fry them in a separate pan for 2 or 3 minutes.

Taste for seasoning, perhaps adding a few drops of fish sauce, a squeeze of fresh lime juice and some freshly chopped coriander.

Serve with the best basmati rice you can find, lightly steamed.

Make a little too much and keep some for tomorrow – it's just that way with curries, they always taste better the next day.

Useful contacts

For cookery classes with Cynthia Mascarenhas
info@namarketing.com 00 44 207 372 0414

YOGA UK
Après Yoga

London
Manna vegetarian restaurant – mannav.com

Norfolk

Norwich
Baba Ghanoush – babaghanoush.co.uk
Café 33, 33 Exchange Street, Norwich NR2 1DP
Sing Sing karaoke bar – singsing.jp
The T Lounge, 143 Ber Street, Norwich NR1 3EY
Tango classes – metrotango.co.uk

Beccles
Fritton House – frittonhouse.co.uk
Somerleyton Hall – somerleyton.co.uk
The Swan House – swan-house.com
Twyfords Café, Exchange Square, Smallgate, Beccles,
    NR34 9HL

Clothes shopping
Anna – shopatanna.co.uk
Collen and Clare – collenandclare.co.uk
Katy's Boutique (a Kiki favourite), 14 Bridewell Alley,
    Norwich, NR2 1AQ
Prim Vintage Fashion (a Kiki favourite), 20 St Benedicts
    St, Norwich NR2 4AQ

Yoga classes
Mandy Brinkley – yellowbeanyoga.co.uk
British Wheel of Yoga Norfolk & Suffolk – yoga-east.org
Annabel Chown – annabelchown@googlemail.com
Dina Cohen – dynamicflow.com
Julee Yew-Crijins – juls.co.uk
Abby Hoffmann – yogawithabby.co.uk
The Life Centre – lifecentre.com
Simon Low holidays & workshops – simonlow.com
Simon Low teacher training – theyogaacademy.org
Claire Missingham – claireyoga.com
triyoga – triyoga.co.uk
Hayley Winter – yogaacademyforsport.co.uk

YOGA INDIA
Drop in centre, Anjuna, Goa – brahmaniyoga.com
Sri K. Pattabhi Jois, Mysore – ayri.org
The Hugging Mother, Kerala – amritapuri.org
Osho, Pune – osho.com
Purple Valley Retreat Centre, Assagao, Goa – yogagoa.com
Sivananda Ashram, Neyyar Dam, Kerala –
    sivananda.org/ndam
Yoga Magic, Anjuna, Goa – yogamagic.net

YOGA SRI LANKA
Ulpotha – ulpotha.com

YOGA USA
Exhale – exhalespa.com
Jivamukti – jivamuktiyoga.com
Shiva Rea – shivarea.com

FERTILITY RESOURCES
Assisted Reproduction & Gynaecology Centre – argc.co.uk
Bourne Hall clinic – bourne-hall-clinic.co.uk
CERAM clinic – ceram.es/ingles
Human Fertilisation and Embryology Authority –
    hfea.gov.uk
Lister Fertility Clinic – ivf.org.uk
Brenda Strong – yoga4fertility.com

GOOD BOOKS ON FERTILITY

Jane English, *Childlessness Transformed: Stories of Alternative Parenting*, Calais, Vermont: Earth Heart, 1989

Sylvia Ann Hewlett, *Creating a Life: What Every Woman Needs to Know About Having a Baby and a Career*, New York: Miramax Books, 2003

Peggy Orenstein, *Waiting for Daisy: The True Story of One Couple's Quest to Have a Baby*, London: Bloomsbury, 2008

Sherman J. Silber, MD, *How to Get Pregnant*, New York: Little Brown & Co., 2007

Acknowledgements

I would like to thank Hannah MacDonald for commissioning this book, Rowan Yapp for her strength of vision, her insight and her utterly rigorous editing and the rest of the team at Ebury, especially Sarah Bennie and Alex Young, Mel Yarker and Anna Derkacz.

Thank you to my agent Araminta Whitley, a compelling combination of steely intelligence, straight talking and dry wit, to Lucy Cowie and the many unsung heroes of LAW for reading early drafts.

Thank you to my friends – you contributed to this book in so many different ways and I owe you all a glass of Pinot Grigio (except Charlie who is eleven): Amy Amos, Mandy Brinkley, Paola de Carolis, Annabel Chown, Rachel Foyer, Alison Glynn, Maria Glynn, Sophie Grenville, Francesca Heathorn, Anne Heigham, Janet Hodgson, Abby Hoffmann, Tiffany Lee, Heather McColm, Ness Merritt, Kerst Morris, Pia Muggerud, Zarmine Sarfaraz Hill, Charlie Satchell, Frances Sinclair, Frances Ruffelle, Liz Walker, Rosie Winston, Hayley Winter, Julee Yew-Crijns.

An especially big thank you to The Bad Ladies for your friendship and willingness to be part of this book – it could not have been written without you.

Thank you BMRB for the yoga statistics.

Thank you to Dr Marie Wren for checking my fertility facts, and for being a brilliant doctor. I hope more women find you through this book.

Thank you to Dorothy Smith for the history of Beccles, to Larry for the jokes, to Alex, Annie, Clare, Frances, Lynda, Michael, Michael, Pansy, Rose, Stuart and Willie for making us so welcome, to Kelly for listening patiently to my weekly updates, to Robin, Jake and Len for unravelling the mysteries of country life for me, and to Father Antony Sutch for having the driest sense of humour and the biggest of hearts.

Finally, to my brothers and sisters, nephews and nieces, Mum and Oliver, Dad and Nikki, Yvonne and Cynthia and the Mascarenhas Diaspora – thank you for all of your love, enthusiasm, patience and support, and to David for your unshakeable belief in me. I love you all more than words can say.

michael newton

Also available by Lucy Edge

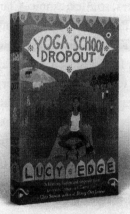

'A hilarious search for a more meaningful life turns
into a joyous discovery of India' *The Times*

'A hilarious, hapless and desperate quest'
Chris Stewart, author of *Driving Over Lemons*

'Lucy Edge, a former London advertising executive goes
in search of spiritual riches (and the perfect headstand) in
India. Neither boringly cynical nor stupidly gullible, she's
open minded, warm and funny; even – though she'd be
the last person to claim this – rather wise'
Independent, Books of the Year

'Fed up with working (and drinking) too much in
advertising [Lucy] heads to India to seek spiritual
enlightenment – and a skinny body and fan club of sweaty,
adoring men while she is at it! Hilarious and wise, discover
whether Lucy manages to find mind opening experiences,
or if true bliss really is a glass of Sauvignon Blanc and
M&S meal for one. Brilliant!' *OK*